Register Now for Online Access to Your Book!

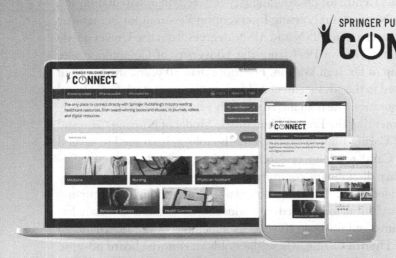

SPRINGER PUBLISHING COMPANY

CONNECT.™

Your print purchase of *An Educator's Guide to Humanizing Nursing Education* **includes online access to the contents of your book**— increasing accessibility, portability, and searchability!

Access today at:

http://connect.springerpub.com/content/book/978-0-8261-9009-3 or scan the QR code at the right with your smartphone and enter the access code below.

Scan here for quick access.

D8YGHCRG

SPRINGER PUBLISHING COMPANY

View all our products at springerpub.com

Chantal Cara, PhD, RN, FAAN, is currently full professor in the Faculty of Nursing, Université de Montréal in Québec, Canada. She is also a researcher at the Montreal's Centre for Interdisciplinary Research in Rehabilitation and at the Quebec Network on Nursing Intervention Research for humanistic practices. She received her BSN and MSN degrees from the Université de Montréal and her PhD in 1997 from the University of Colorado, under the directorship of Dr. Jean Watson. For more than 30 years, she has been actively involved in the advancement of Human Caring in both French and English communities. She is an internationally renowned scholar for creating and implementing the French Humanistic Model of Nursing Care and the Relational Caring Inquiry research methodology, both used in several countries. Dr. Cara's teaching, research activities, publications, and conferences reflect her disciplinary commitment to disseminate internationally her theory-guided research findings aimed at fostering humanistic nursing practices in the clinical, managerial, and educational domains. Dr. Cara has been actively involved for over 20 years as a member of the International Association of Human Caring, where she holds an editorial board position on the *International Journal for Human Caring*. She is vice president of the Global Alliance for Human Caring Education (2018–). She is also a reviewer for the *Advances in Nursing Science* as well as an international advisory board member of the editorial board for the scientific journal *Health SA Gesondheid* published in South Africa. Since 2015, she has been an invited professor/caring scholar at the University of Colorado, and at the Institut et Haute École La Source, Switzerland. In 2016, she was the first to be attributed the title Distinguished Watson Caring Science Scholar by the Watson Caring Science Institute. In 2018, she was the first in Quebec to be inducted as a fellow of the American Academy of Nursing.

Marcia Hills, PhD, RN, FAAN, is a professor at the School of Nursing, Faculty of Human and Social Development, University of Victoria, British Columbia, Canada. She was the founding director of the British Columbia Collaborative Nursing Program—the first Caring Science nursing program in Canada (1989–1994); founding director of the Centre for Community Health Promotion Research (2002–2009) at the University of Victoria; cochair (2002–2004) and then president (2004–2008) of the Canadian Consortium for Health Promotion Research (CCHPR); president of the Canadian Association of Teachers for Community Health (CATCH; 2004–2015); and a globally elected member of the Board of Trustees of the International Union for Health Promotion and Education (IUHPE; 2001–2013) and vice president for research and technical development (2010–2013) and cochair of the Health Promotion Effectiveness Project (2005–2009) of its North

American region. She is a distinguished scholar of Caring Science and faculty associate at the Watson Caring Science Institute (WCSI) and was the inaugural chair of its Faculty Executive and Faculty Council (2010–2014) and the academic lead of its WCSI Doctoral Program. Dr. Hills is the founder and current president of the Global Alliance for Human Caring Education (2018–). She coauthored, with Dr. Jean Watson (2011), *Creating a Caring Science Curriculum: An Emancipatory Pedagogy for Nursing* and currently is working on its second edition. As a visiting scholar and a World Health Organization (WHO) fellow, Dr. Hills worked and studied in Australia, England, and Brazil, at the National School of Public Health in Rio de Janeiro. She has consulted extensively in the United States, the United Kingdom, New Zealand, Australia, Trinidad and Tobago, Kenya, Brazil, Chile, and Canada in the areas of health promotion, primary healthcare, emancipatory caring curriculum development and pedagogy, women's health, and participatory action research and evaluation.

Jean Watson, PhD, RN, AHN-BC, FAAN, LL-AAN, is distinguished professor and dean emerita, University of Colorado College of Nursing Anschutz Medical Center. She is the founder of the original Center for Human Caring in Colorado, a fellow of the American Academy of Nursing (FAAN), the founder and director of the nonprofit organization Watson Caring Science Institute, and the past president of the National League for Nursing. Dr. Watson is also a founding member of the International Association for Human Caring and the International Caritas Consortium. She held the nation's first endowed chair in Caring Science for 16 years. She holds 15 honorary doctoral degrees, including 12 international honorary doctorates. Her work is studied and implemented around the world. She is a widely published author and recipient of many awards and honors; she has authored and coauthored over 30 books on caring. In October 2013, Dr. Watson was inducted as a Living Legend by the American Academy of Nursing—its highest honor.

An Educator's Guide to Humanizing Nursing Education

Grounded in Caring Science

Chantal Cara, PhD, RN, FAAN

Marcia Hills, PhD, RN, FAAN

*Jean Watson, PhD, RN, AHN-BC,
FAAN, LL-AAN*

SPRINGER PUBLISHING COMPANY

Springer Publishing Company, LLC
11 West 42nd Street, New York, NY 10036
www.springerpub.com
http://connect.springerpub.com/home

Acquisitions Editor: Adrianne Brigido
Compositor: Amnet Systems

ISBN: 978-0-8261-9008-6
ebook ISBN: 978-0-8261-9009-3
DOI: 10.1891/9780826190093

20 21 22 23 24 / 5 4 3 2 1

The author and the publisher of this Work have made every effort to use sources believed to be reliable to provide information that is accurate and compatible with the standards generally accepted at the time of publication. The author and publisher shall not be liable for any special, consequential, or exemplary damages resulting, in whole or in part, from the readers' use of, or reliance on, the information contained in this book. The publisher has no responsibility for the persistence or accuracy of URLs for external or third-party Internet websites referred to in this publication and does not guarantee that any content on such websites is, or will remain, accurate or appropriate.

Library of Congress Cataloging-in-Publication Data

Names: Cara, Chantal, author. | Hills, Marcia, author. | Watson, Jean, author.
Title: An educator's guide to humanizing nursing education : grounded in caring science / Chantal Cara, Marcia Hills, Jean Watson.
Description: New York, NY : Springer Publishing Company, LLC, [2021] | Includes bibliographical references and index.
Identifiers: LCCN 2020005080 (print) | LCCN 2020005081 (ebook) | ISBN 9780826190086 (paperback) | ISBN 9780826190093 (ebook)
Subjects: MESH: Education, Nursing | Philosophy, Nursing | Teaching | Empathy
Classification: LCC RT71 (print) | LCC RT71 (ebook) | NLM WY 18 | DDC 610.73071—dc23
LC record available at https://lccn.loc.gov/2020005080
LC ebook record available at https://lccn.loc.gov/2020005081

Contact us to receive discount rates on bulk purchases.
We can also customize our books to meet your needs.
For more information please contact: sales@springerpub.com

Publisher's Note: New and used products purchased from third-party sellers are not guaranteed for quality, authenticity, or access to any included digital components.

Printed in the United States of America.

*To the memory of my dear colleagues and mentors,
Dr. Georgette Desjean, Thérèse Doucet, and Suzanne Kérouac,
who contributed to introducing Human Caring at
the Université de Montréal.
My gratitude to both Jean and Marcia for their teaching
and support over the years and for accepting to be part of this
project with me.
To my husband, John, and
my lovely daughters, Stéphany and Émily,
whose enduring support and presence allowed me to fulfill
my Human Caring journey.
To them, my deepest gratitude for their unconditional love.*
—Chantal Cara

*Whenever I participate in advancing Caring Science,
I am compelled to dedicate my work to Em Bevis and Jean Watson.
They introduced me to this Caring Science journey,
and although Em has now passed away, she remains with
me on this journey! Jean continues to mentor and challenge
me to create my legacy, and it is with her encouragement that
I entered this project.
Also, I dedicate this work to all my students
who have taught me so much about Caring Science and
how to humanize nursing education. Thank you,
Chantal, for inviting me to join in this rewarding endeavor.*
—Marcia Hills

*To all the students and colleagues over these years
who have taught me the significance of honoring them and
their inner life-world as a sacred trust and
the only source for true learning.*
—Jean Watson

Contents

Contributors

Houssem Eddine Ben Ahmed, PhD(c), MSc, RN
  Doctoral Student and Teaching Assistant
  Faculty of Nursing, Université de Montréal
  Montréal, Québec, Canada

Sylvain Brousseau, PhD, MSc, BSN, RN
  Associate Professor in Nursing Science and Director of the
  Undergraduate Nursing Science program
  Université du Québec en Outaouais
  Saint-Jérôme, Québec, Canada

Jessica Eitel, MN, BSN, RNC-NIC
  Research Nurse Coordinator
  University of British Columbia, BC Children's Hospital
  Vancouver, British Columbia, Canada
  Neonatal Nursing Instructor
  Mount Royal University Continuing Education
  Calgary, Alberta, Canada

Benita Lee, MN, BScN, RN, CPN(C)
  Clinical Nurse, Operating Room
  The Hospital for Sick Children
  Toronto, Ontario, Canada

Dimitri Létourneau, PhD, RN
  Assistant Professor
  Faculty of Nursing, Université de Montréal
  Montréal, Québec, Canada

Colleen Maykut, DNP, MN, BScN, RN
Associate Professor
MacEwan University
Faculty of Nursing—Department of Nursing Science
Edmonton, Alberta, Canada

Cole Miller, BScN, RN
Registered Nurse
Grey Nuns Community Hospital—Emergency Department
Edmonton, Alberta, Canada

Louise O'Reilly, PhD, MSc, RN
Adjunct Professor, School of Nursing, Université de Sherbrooke
Sherbrooke, Québec, Canada
Adjunct Professor, Faculty of Nursing, Université de Montréal
Montréal, Québec, Canada

Amélie Ouellet, MSc, RN
Lecturer, School of Nursing, Université de Sherbrooke
Nurse Clinician, Department of Intellectual Disabilities and
Autism Spectrum Disorders
Centre intégré universitaire de santé et de services sociaux de l'Estrie
Centre hospitalier universitaire de Sherbrooke
Sherbrooke, Québec, Canada

Ruhina Rana, MN, BSN, BA, RN
Health Sciences Research Coordinator
Faculty, Bachelor of Science Nursing
Douglas College
Vancouver, British Columbia, Canada

Nancy J. Vitali, DCS, MS, RN
Associate Professor of Nursing (Retired)
Tulsa Community College
Adjunct Professor of Nursing
Oklahoma University College of Nursing
Tulsa, Oklahoma, United States

M. Carol Wild, MScN, RN
Area Manager
Ponoka Hospital & Care Centre
Alberta Health Services
Ponoka, Alberta, Canada

Zane Robinson Wolf, PhD, RN, CNE, FAAN
Dean Emerita, Adjunct Professor
La Salle University, School of Nursing and Health Sciences
Philadelphia, Pennsylvania, United States

Foreword

To our precious students:

> Your journey is our journey, your future is ours. How you are prepared
> to join, and perhaps lead a community, a generation, a world, matters
> to those who have gone before you and those who will come after you.
> —Cathy N. Davidson, *The New Education*, 2017, p. 2

Educating nurses is a sacred and serious undertaking. Those of us who dedicate our lives to this calling understand that we are charged with preparing the next generation of nurses to accept the profound responsibilities for the health, well-becoming, and healing of people they will serve. We know that the educational journey in our discipline is not merely one of providing the knowledge and skills necessary to practice in the profession. It is about facilitating growth from the inside out. We educate nurses for praxis, the integration of knowing–doing–being in service to others. We are privileged to witness the inner transformation from student to nurse, like the miracle of a seed growing and blossoming into a beautiful flower. This inner journey is the hero's journey, described by Joseph Campbell (1949) as having three phases: the departure, the initiation, and the return. It is a journey of hearing a call, crossing a threshold into the unfamiliar, encountering challenges that seem insurmountable, discovering unimaginable strengths and gifts within the self, and returning to share these gifts with others. The mentor or guide is a sojourner, charting the path, encouraging, supporting, bearing witness to struggles, and celebrating successes. This is the way of the teacher on the educational journey.

Unfortunately, there are many barriers to this vision of teaching/learning. The business model emphasizing conformity, productivity, cost-effectiveness, and prescriptive outcomes drives educators to move students through a system expeditiously. In nursing education, the emphasis on passing licensing

and certification exams often eclipses the importance of self-reflection and
self-care. The teaching/learning processes in most educational systems
emphasize control over freedom, conformity over creativity, power-over
instead of empowerment, and objectivity over engagement. And yet we
know that these dehumanizing processes thwart the ability to prepare the
next generation for the challenges of the 21st century, and most definitely
are barriers to preparing nurses for their future caring–healing praxis.

Nurse educators are role models. Students learn ways of being-with
others from their experiences in the teaching/learning environment. This
environment is fertile ground for cultivating a myriad of ontological gifts
such as presence, authenticity, nurturance, compassion, appreciating differences, courage, and learning from mistakes. Students grow in caring through
experiencing caring with those who engage with them in the teaching/
learning process. When educators truly walk with students on this educational journey—coming to know them, encouraging reflection, providing
safe space for exploring thoughts, feelings, and perceptions, and nurturing
their growth—students internalize this way of being-with others. Similarly,
teachers often learn to teach from how they were taught. There is an urgent
need for educators to learn a different pedagogy. There is an urgent need
for an educational revolution in nursing toward an emancipatory pedagogy.
Kagan, Smith, and Chinn (2016) define emancipatory processes as disrupting
structural inequities, facilitating humanization, promoting self-reflection,
and engaging communities.

*An Educator's Guide to Humanizing Nursing Education: Grounded in Caring
Science* is an inspired book with the ingredients needed for this emancipatory
educational revolution. The book is authored by experts in the pedagogy of
Caring Science. They are scholars extraordinaire who have practiced this
pedagogy and understand the miracles that can happen when it is lived in the
teaching/learning environment. Dr. Chantal Cara, professor, Caring Science
scholar, and dynamic international nursing leader, developed a humanistic
model of care that has informed the work presented in this book. Dr. Marcia
Hills, master educator and Caring Science scholar, has focused her life's
work on caring pedagogy. Dr. Jean Watson, acclaimed theorist and nursing
legend, inspired both Drs. Cara and Hills and continues to seed the work of
many scholars around the world. Most of the contributors to the Pragmatic
Segments of the chapters are Canadian and have been engaged in teaching
from a humanistic, relational, emancipatory philosophical perspective. They
share the fruits of their rich experiences in these chapters.

The chapters in this book build from the abstract foundations to the
specific examples, leading to an integration of knowledge and a call to action.
The first chapter provides the necessary foundation in a human science

paradigm that has the promise to address the challenges in nursing education. The next chapter moves to the more explicit values and attitudes from a Caring Science model that contributes to the humanization of nursing education. Chapter 3 focuses on emancipatory philosophy and its possibilities for nursing education. Chapter 4 gives meaning to nurse educators' practice of "teaching from the heart," and Chapter 5 informs them on how to foster caring teaching/learning relationships with their students. The following chapters provide specificity and clarity, providing language and exemplars from Watson's Caritas Processes and other literacies that offer substantive directions for a paradigm shift in nursing education.

This text is an essential resource for all nurses interested in or engaged in education. As an emancipatory text, it evokes informed action. For those already aware of the need for educational reform, it will provide support and new ideas needed to advance your work. For those new to these concepts, this book will be the spark to ignite your participation in the transformation of nursing education. I am grateful to the authors and contributors for this brilliant text and anticipate the difference it will make in Caring Science pedagogy, the praxis of future nurses, and the health, well-becoming, and healing of those we serve.

Marlaine C. Smith, PhD, RN, AHN-BC, HWNC-BC, FAAN
Professor and Helen K. Persson Eminent Scholar
Christine E. Lynn College of Nursing, Florida Atlantic University

REFERENCES

Campbell, J. (1949). *The hero with a thousand faces*. New York, NY: Pantheon Books.

Davidson, C. N. (2017). *The new education: How to revolutionize the university to prepare students for a world in flux*. New York, NY: Basic Books.

Kagan, P. N, Smith, M. C., & Chinn, P. L. (2016). *Philosophies and practices of emancipatory nursing: Social justice as praxis*. New York, NY: Routledge.

Preface

This book was written in response to a darker aspect of nursing education: dehumanizing practices toward students and the impacts such practices may have on both students and their learning. Hence, it offers guidance on how to be inspired by Human Caring to overcome such challenges to humanize nursing education and ground the nurse educator's role in developing authentic caring teaching/learning relationships with students. Our goal in writing this book was that it should be beneficial to nurse educators, teachers, professors, Caritas Coaches, as well as graduate students studying nursing education to enlighten their caring–teaching practices.

This book assists in translating caring values, attitudes, and behaviors into knowing, doing, being, and becoming caring nurse educators to uphold the importance of the relational nature of their work with students. It explains how Human Caring can expand nurse educators' consciousness to explore the path to a Relational Emancipatory Pedagogy for nursing education. This book also gives meaning to nurse educators' practice of "teaching from the heart," a primary raison d'être, contributing to make a difference in students' lives.

It also shares how Caritas Processes and Caritas Literacy can inform nurse educators in their daily teaching/learning practices. This text explains how a caring worldview may enhance nurse educators' moral imperative to develop and foster "habitus," an ontological space, to enable students to explore healing as their professional purpose. Additionally, this book aims to elucidate how nurse educators can influence their nursing school colleagues and workforce politically to shape the relationships within the institution, contributing to humanizing nursing education.

Each chapter includes learning intentions, a theoretical segment, some "Time Out for Reflection" segments to foster the integration of theory into practice, as well as a Pragmatic Segment. Overall, those Pragmatic Segments correspond to a wealth of case examples provided by administrators, nurse educators, and students to illustrate the value of a humanistic paradigm for nursing education and caring pedagogical praxis. Finally, this book intends to enlighten nurse educators to accompany their students in their learning journey, inspiring their reflective practice and opening toward a dialogical discussion. Ultimately, this book offers a new lens and a new *Being-Caring* perspective of teaching as a new mandate for nursing education.

Chantal Cara
Marcia Hills
Jean Watson

Acknowledgments

We want to acknowledge all of our precious contributors for agreeing to participate in our book. By sharing their stories, they have all contributed to illustrate the value of Human Caring in nursing education.

We wish to express our deepest gratitude to Dr. Marlaine Smith, a great Caring Science scholar, for accepting our invitation to write the foreword of this book.

Our appreciation extends to all our colleagues from the International Association for Human Caring and the Watson Caring Science Institute, as well as all our nurse educators, colleagues, and graduate students for their ongoing efforts to advance the work of Human Caring in all domains of the discipline of nursing.

Lastly, we would like to acknowledge the essential work of M. John Hills. Our deepest gratitude to him for his precious voluntary editing of most of the chapters in this book. His careful and meticulous reviewing and editing were invaluable.

1

Grounded in a Human Science Paradigm: Human Caring to Overcome Challenges to Humanize Nursing Education

For nursing students, who enter educational programs primarily to care for others, uncaring encounters may be extremely detrimental for them as individuals. . . . If nursing education programs do not fundamentally aspire to actualizing caring encounters, learning may be sabotaged, leading to inappropriate and/or a lack of understanding of the importance of caring as the foundation of nursing.
—Adams and Maykut, 2015, p. 768

LEARNING INTENTIONS

- Sensitize nurse educators about the impact of dehumanizing teaching practices on students and their learning.
- Reflect on how Human Caring can overcome dehumanizing teaching practices in order to humanize nursing education.

1

- Appreciate how Human Caring can promote students' learning and foster their caring praxis.
- Understand, from students' perspective, how dehumanizing teaching practices can impede their learning and success.

INTRODUCTION

We first acknowledge a darker aspect of nursing education: nurse educators' dehumanizing practices toward students. After explaining this unfortunate, yet frequent, phenomenon and its impact on both the students and their learning, we discuss the importance of Human Caring in overcoming such challenges in order to humanize nursing education and ground the educator's role, and the teaching/learning relationships. We introduce the added value of caring relationships for students and nurse educators alike, and we present our philosophical foundation to support our Human Caring approach as a cornerstone to enhance humanization in nursing education. A Pragmatic Segment will illustrate these ideas more concretely.

WHY WE NEED TO HUMANIZE NURSING EDUCATION

Dehumanizing practices are no longer just studied or addressed in clinical nursing, but they are also prevalent in nursing education. In fact, there are some authors who are beginning to discuss dehumanizing practices in nursing education.

According to Haslam (2006), dehumanizing practices appear in academic domains mostly because of the prevalence of standardized assessment and teaching practices, "which are rigid and impersonal and treat students as passive and uncreative" (p. 254). Hills and Cara (2019) explain that the traditional behaviorist paradigm, which considers nurse educators as the experts teaching the only desirable behaviors to be evaluated, may contribute to such educational practices. Indeed, this behaviorist perspective fails to recognize the uniqueness and diversity of students and their learning processes; does not consider an interactive and heuristic approach to students' learning; and, most importantly, does not acknowledge the importance of the student–educator relationship in their learning.

In nursing education literature, such dehumanization is given different labels, including uncaring behaviors, unethical attitudes, incivility, bullying, abuse, harassment, as well as horizontal and lateral violence (see Table 1.1). In this book, we use the term *dehumanizing teaching practices*.

Table 1.1 **Different Concepts or Constructs Used in the Nursing Literature**

Constructs Used	Authors
Uncaring behaviors	Cara and Hills (2018)
Uncaring encounters	Halldorsdottir (1990)
Incivility	Beck (2015); Muliira, Natarajan, and van der Colff (2017); Ziefle (2018)
Bullying	Adams and Maykut (2015); Birks, Budden, Stewart, and Chapman (2014); Seibel and Fehr (2018); Stagg, Sheridan, Jones, and Speroni (2013)
Abuse	Stagg et al. (2013)
Harassment	Birks et al. (2014)
Horizontal and lateral violence	Hills and Watson (2011); Seibel and Fehr (2018); Thomas (2010)
Unethical attitudes	Arslan and Dinç (2017)

Although contemporary literature addresses reciprocal dehumanizing practices (both nurse educators toward students and students toward nurse educators), in this book, we concentrate on nurse educators' dehumanizing teaching practices toward students. An example of such dehumanizing practices in nursing education could be a nurse educator humiliating his or her students in front of classmates in the classroom or in front of patients, family members, nurses, physicians, or other healthcare professionals during their clinical practicum.

Dehumanization: Understanding the Phenomenon

Dehumanization, in general, has been discussed mostly in relation to healthcare and organizations. According to Christoff (2014) and Haslam (2006) who are both from the field of psychology, "dehumanization" is defined as the fact that a person is being objectified or considered as an object. Moreover, it often occurs with indifference, a lack of empathy, along with an abstract and stigmatized view of the person (Haslam, 2006). In their study with rehabilitation patients, dehumanization has also been associated with work overload, bureaucracy, lack of time, and a task-oriented approach (Avoine, 2012; Avoine, O'Reilly, & Michaud, 2012; Avoine, O'Reilly, Michaud, & St-Cyr Tribble, 2011).

Considering more closely the expression "uncaring encounters," Halldorsdottir's work (1990, 1991, 2013) can be extremely valuable to understand dehumanization, dehumanizing practices, as well as their damaging impacts on the person. She describes "uncaring encounters" as corresponding especially to three modes of being with another. She refers to the first one, the "life-destroying (biocidic) mode of being with another" (see Table 1.2), as the most inhumane encounter (Halldorsdottir, 2013, p. 202). This is a "mode where one depersonalizes the other, destroys the joy of life, and increases the other's vulnerability. It causes distress, despair and hurts and deforms the other. It is transference of negative energy and darkness" (Halldorsdottir, 2013, p. 202). This author explains that this particular uncaring encounter mode is characterized by numerous manifestations of inhumane attitudes by the nurse, for example, aggression, manipulation, humiliation, dominance, coercion, and depersonalization. According to Halldorsdottir, the person's reaction can range from puzzlement and disbelief, to anger and resentment, to helplessness and despair. For example, in nursing education, an educator could humiliate a student in front of her or his colleagues for failing an assignment.

Halldorsdottir (2013) explains the second mode, the "life-restraining (biostatic) mode of being with another" (see Table 1.2), as a "mode where one is insensitive or indifferent to the other and detached from the true center of the other. It causes discouragement and develops uneasiness in the other. It negatively affects existing life in the other" (p. 202). According to this author, this second type of uncaring encounter entails forcing one's own will and dominating and controlling the other person. Moreover, during such an uncaring encounter, Halldorsdottir (2013) describes that the nurse's presence is considered as disruptive as exhibiting rudeness and lack of kindness. For example, in nursing education, in wanting to display better knowledge of the course and its contents, sometimes nurse educators could show a bitter response and discourage or even fail a student simply for having a different point of view than theirs.

Halldorsdottir (2013) explicates that the third mode, "life-neutral, or biopassive, mode of being with another" (see Table 1.2), takes place "when one is detached from the true center of the other and when there is no effect on the energy or life of the other. This lack of response, interest, and affect derives from inattentiveness or insensitivity" (p. 205). Although there is no tangible effect on the person's life, Halldorsdottir argues that such uncaring encounters may often create a feeling of loneliness from the absence of relationships. For example, in nursing education, educators could be insensitive to their students' difficulties in the classroom and may not want to connect and accompany them to foster their learning.

Dehumanization corresponds to the fact of being treated as an object with an obvious lack of respect. It also implies being deprived of one's own

Table 1.2 Dehumanization From Halldorsdottir's Mode of Being With Another

Halldorsdottir's Mode of Being With Another	Nurses' Attitudes	Consequences for the Person
Life-destroying (biocidic)	Aggression Manipulation Humiliation Domination Coercion Depersonalization	Vulnerability Suffering Distress Despair Anger Resentment Helplessness
Life-restraining (biostatic)	Insensitivity Indifference Disruptive Controlling Rudeness	Affecting negatively Discouragement Uneasiness
Life-neutral (biopassive)	Lack of response Lack of interest Inattentiveness Insensitivity	Loneliness from the absence of relationships

Source: Adapted from Halldorsdottir, S. (2013). Five basic modes of being with another. In M. C. Smith, M. C. Turkel, & Z. R. Wolf (Eds.), *Caring in nursing classics. An essential resource* (pp. 201–210). New York, NY: Springer Publishing Company.

human dignity and personhood—no longer being acknowledged as a human being—which may amplify one's frustrations, vulnerability, suffering, and despair.

Several authors have identified various nurse educators' dehumanizing practices, such as:

- Exhibiting rigidity
- Rudeness
- Disparaging feedback
- Avoidance
- Unethical action
- Racism
- Condescension
- Favoritism
- Discrimination
- Objectification (Adams & Maykut, 2015; Arslan & Dinç, 2017; Beck, 2015; Cara & Hills, 2018; Muliira, Natarajan, & van der Colff, 2017; Seibel & Fehr, 2018; Ziefle, 2018).

According to Christoff (2014), there are various levels of dehumanization, ranging anywhere from mild and subtle (e.g., subtle disrespect and condescension) to obvious and severe (e.g., neglect and social ostracism). As Arslan and Dinç (2017) explain,

> the teacher–student relationship is inherently one of power, based on teachers' professional knowledge, skills, and authority and students' dependence. Power and position asymmetry within this relationship creates the potential for the mistreatment, abuse and exploitation of students, negatively influencing students' formal socialization and the effectiveness of education. (p. 790)

These nurse educators' dehumanizing practices may generate various emotions in students such as anxiety, stress, and powerlessness (see Table 1.3). Christoff (2014) explains that dehumanization, in general, can leave a person feeling angry, degraded, incompetent, excluded, and not recognized as a human being.

Table 1.3 Examples of Students' Responses to Nurse Educators' Dehumanizing Practices and Their Impacts

Students' Responses	Impacts
Anxiety	Decreased learning
Stress	Depression
Humiliation	Suffering
Powerlessness	Attrition
Distress	Failure

Sources: Data from Adams, L. Y., & Maykut, C. (2015). Bullying: The antithesis of caring acknowledging the dark side of the nursing profession. *International Journal for Caring Sciences, 8*(3), 765–773. Retrieved from http://www.internationaljournalofcaringsciences.org/docs/28_Adams_special_8_3.pdf; Arslan, S., & Dinç, L. (2017). Nursing students' perceptions of faculty members' ethical/unethical attitudes. *Nursing Ethics, 24*(7), 789–801. doi:10.1177/0969733015625366; Beck, D. M. (2015). Incivility and student and faculty relationships: Implications for revising mentorship programs for nurse educators. *SOJ Nursing & Health Care, 1*(1), 1–10. doi:10.15226/2471-6529/1/1/00103; Cara, C., & Hills, M. (2018, May). *The added value of Caring Science: Its contributions to humanize nursing education.* Oral presentation, Canadian Association of Schools in Nursing (CASN) Conference, Montreal, QC, Canada; Muliira, J. K., Natarajan, J., & van der Colff, J. (2017). Nursing faculty academic incivility: Perceptions of nursing students and faculty. *BMC Medical Education, 17*(1), 1–10. doi:10.1186/s12909-017-1096-8; Seibel, L. M., & Fehr, F. C. (2018). "They can crush you": Nursing students' experiences of bullying and the role of faculty. *Journal of Nursing Education and Practice, 8*(6), 66–76. doi:10.5430/jnep.v8n6p66; Ziefle, K. (2018). Incivility in nursing education: Generational differences. *Teaching and Learning in Nursing, 13*(1), 27–30. doi:10.1016/j.teln.2017.09.004.

Numerous authors have highlighted different impacts or consequences of dehumanizing practices for students, such as decreased learning, suffering, and failure (see Table 1.3). In fact, according to Seibel and Fehr (2018), "unaddressed bullying can lead to deeper issues such as entrenched negative behaviour. . . . Students and new graduates leave the profession due to bullying" (p. 70).

Such impacts should be a huge concern for nurse educators. To quote Adams and Maykut (2015),

> uncaring encounters occur . . . speaking about the dark side is necessary; we can no longer pretend it doesn't exist or is inconsequential. . . . Addressing bullying, as an uncaring encounter, will ensure that as nurses we are able to accomplish the mandate of caring and protecting our patients. (p. 771)

TIME OUT FOR REFLECTION

The authors invite you to write your reflection in a journal in order to link the preceding theoretical segment with your personal teaching/learning experiences.

Think about a time when you were in a situation where it felt dehumanizing, and then ask yourself the following questions:
- Who was involved?
- What were the characteristics illustrating dehumanization?
- What was your lived experience?
- How did you feel?
- What were you telling yourself at the time?
- What were the impacts at a personal level?
- What were the impacts for your teaching/learning practices?
- What solutions did you consider at the time to rehumanize the situation?
- Could it have been different? Explain briefly.

HUMANIZING NURSING EDUCATION

One way to shift from dehumanizing to humanizing nursing education is by adopting a humanist perspective. In general, such a perspective places emphasis on people, their experiences, their meanings, and their relationships (Cara, 2017; Cara & Hills, 2018). In a nursing education context, a humanist perspective would, therefore, focus on the students, their learning experiences, their meanings, and their relationships (Cara & Hills, 2018).

Humanist philosophers, such as Buber (1970/1996), Rogers (1961), and Mayeroff (1971/1990), have several beliefs in common. They

> all considered humans' growth as a central component of their work. In fact, they clearly stated that human development is enhanced through a relationship, nurtured by both persons involved. These authors also shared a similar belief about authenticity (or congruence), understood as a quality of the relationship and as a prerequisite for its establishment. (Létourneau, Cara, & Goudreau, 2017, p. 34)

In fact, these humanist philosophers have served as an underpinning for several caring theories in nursing, such as those of Watson (1985/1988, 2008, 2012), Roach (1984, 2002), Boykin and Schoenhofer (1993, 1993/2001), as well as Cara et al. (2016), mainly because of their emphasis on concepts such as "relationship" and "growth." Furthermore, a humanist perspective is grounded in humanistic values, such as respect and human dignity, suggesting that nurse educators should rethink the importance of preserving their students' human dignity when dealing, for example, with learning difficulties and failures (see also Chapter 2, Educators' Caring Values, Attitudes, and Behaviors That Contribute to the Humanization of Nursing Education).

Therefore, Human Caring could contribute to rehumanize nursing education by inviting nurse educators to focus on their relationships with students and nurture students' professional growth, by accompanying them to become the best nurses possible.

Human Caring in Nursing Education

"Caring Science provides this deep underpinning for a scientific-philosophical-moral context from which to explore, describe, and research human caring–healing phenomena . . . that informs and inspires the discipline and profession of nursing" (Hills & Watson, 2011, p. 12). In other words, Human Caring provides a disciplinary foundation comprising science, ontology, and ethics to guide nurse educators to humanize nursing education. By "ontology," we mean the nature of being, our existence, as well as the reality. Hence, as many have suggested (Bevis & Watson, 1989/2000; Boykin, Touhy, & Smith, 2011; Hills & Watson, 2011), nursing education programs would gain from being based on a clear moral, theoretical, and philosophical foundation, such as Human Caring. Such a perspective would then inform teachers on how to become a caring nurse educator, being one's moral imperative.

We can then ask the question, What does it mean to be/become a caring nurse educator? To be/become a caring nurse educator is to develop humanist relationships with students in order to promote their learning, their personal meaning, and their dignity (Cara & Hills, 2018). Developing a caring pedagogical relationship requires interactions between the nurse educators and their student(s) that are respectful, authentic, humanist, and are based on equity, trust, and safety (see Chapter 5, Seeking Teaching/Learning Caring Relationships With Students). Consequently, the student–educator relationship is fundamental, but a caring nurse educator's main goal is not solely the relationship in itself, but rather primarily, the students' learning. Indeed, a nurse educator, inspired by a Human Caring approach, will accompany students in their learning of what nursing is and ought to be, in order for them to find their learning meaningful.

Several authors have acknowledged the importance of student–educator relationships in students' learning (Boykin, Touhy, & Smith, 2011; Cara et al., 2016; Cara & Hills, 2018; Chan, Tong, & Henderson, 2017; Froneman, Du Plessis, & Koen, 2016; Hills & Cara, 2019; Hills & Watson, 2011; Labrague, McEnroe-Petitte, Papathanasiou, Edet, & Arulappan, 2015; Noddings, 2013; Smith & Crowe, 2017; Whealan, 2017). "One of the most important factors influencing education quality and effectiveness is teacher-student interaction" (Arslan & Dinç, 2017, p. 790). In other words, student–educator relationships are ontologically fundamental to students' learning. Nurse educators' caring ontology, acknowledging the relational aspect of teaching as central for students' learning, will guide them to being and becoming caring educators.

Added Value for Students and Nurse Educators

Whealan (2017) acknowledges the importance of caring in nursing education. "From an educator's perspective, helping students develop caring literacy is a moral imperative because caring is the very essence of nursing. How we, as educators, instill and nurture caring among students is vital" (p. 40).

Several authors and researchers have highlighted the added value of the student–educator relationship for students—decreased anxiety, feeling more confident and resilient, feeling empowered, and so forth (see Table 1.4). Several authors have also recognized the overall contribution to students' general learning to improve their caring practices for their patients in clinical settings (see Table 1.4).

In contrast, only a few authors and researchers have highlighted the added value of the student–educator relationship for nurse educators (see Table 1.5).

Table 1.4 Added Values of Student–Educator Relationships for Students

Added Values for Students	Authors
Decreased anxiety	Chan, Tong, and Henderson (2017)
Feeling respected	Beck (2001); Chan et al. (2017); Gillespie (2005); Halldorsdottir (1990); Miller, Harber, and Byrne (1990)
Feeling more confident and resilient	Beck (2001); Froneman, Du Plessis, and Koen (2016); Labrague, McEnroe-Petitte, Papathanasiou, Edet, and Arulappan (2015)
Feeling empowered	Beck (2001); Hills and Watson (2011); Miller et al. (1990)
Growth and transformation	Beck (2001); Gillespie (2005); Halldorsdottir (1990); Hills and Watson (2011); Miller et al. (1990)
Increased general learning	Beck (2001); Cara et al. (2016); Chan et al. (2017); Froneman et al. (2016); Gillespie (2005); Halldorsdottir (1990); Hills and Watson (2011); Labrague et al. (2015)
Improved clinical caring practices	Beck (2001); Cara et al. (2016); Chan et al. (2017); Froneman et al. (2016); Gillespie (2005); Halldorsdottir (1990); Hills and Watson (2011); Labrague et al. (2015)

Table 1.5 Added Values of Student–Educator Relationships for Nurse Educators

Added Values for Nurse Educators	Authors
Hope for the future of nursing	Miller, Haber, and Byrne (1990)
Holistic concerns for their students	Beck (2001); Miller et al. (1990)
Enthusiasm for teaching	Chan, Tong, and Henderson (2017)
Professional growth	Gillespie (2005); Miller et al. (1990)
Well-being	Froneman, Du Plessis, and Koen (2016)
Overall quality of the education offered	Froneman et al. (2016)

TIME OUT FOR REFLECTION

The authors invite you to write your reflection in a journal in order to link the preceding theoretical segment with your personal teaching/learning experiences.

Think about a time when you were in a situation where it felt humanizing for yourself and your student. Again, ask yourself these questions:

- Who was involved?
- What were the characteristics reflecting the humanization?
- What was your lived experience like?
- How did you feel?
- What were you telling yourself at the time?
- What were the advantages for your student?
- What were the advantages for yourself and in your teaching/learning practices?

HUMAN CARING WITHIN A HUMAN SCIENCE PARADIGM

Historically, most nursing programs have been based in an orthodox, positivistic, and behavioral paradigm (Bevis & Watson, 1989/2000; Hills & Watson, 2011; National League for Nursing [NLN], 1988, 2003) or, as Zander and Zander (2002) label it, a "world of measurement." This worldview has an ontology of separation and compartmentalization. It attempts to be neutral but actually values objectivity and is reductionistic. This empiricist worldview uses an objectivist–empirical epistemology to understand the world through probability statistics and suggests that everything can and must be measured (Hills & Watson, 2011). It embraces an experimental methodology typically using large datasets and scientifically controlled procedures. As Reason (1994) explains,

> orthodox research methods, as part of their rationale, exclude human subjects from all the thinking and decision-making that generates and designs, manages and draws conclusions, from the research. Such exclusions treat the subjects as less than self-determining persons, alienate them from the inquiry process and from the knowledge that is its outcome, and thus invalidates any claim the methods have to a science of persons. (p. 280)

By contrast, Human Caring is situated in a Human Science paradigm, which has a relational ontology that values subjectivity and peoples' experiences (Hills & Watson, 2011; Watson, 2012). This Human Science paradigm values multiple ways of knowing and knowledge and uses an expanded pluralistic epistemology to understand the world. It seeks understanding of meaning and peoples' experiences using multiple methodologies such as narrative inquiry, phenomenology, ethnography, and artistic methods.

Locating nursing education in this Human Science paradigm requires a shift in thinking, being, and doing that holds people and our humanity at the center of our educational practice. This means what educators say and do and the way that they are ("their being") is paramount in every interaction and transaction with their students. It lays the

> foundation for reconnecting the heart, soul, mind, emotions, and the human spirit of students and teachers alike; it invites passion, intellect, moral ideals, and love into our classrooms and curriculum, restoring humanity and human caring–healing knowledge and practices for now and the future. (Hills & Watson, 2011, p. 16)

PRAGMATIC SEGMENT
HINDRANCE TO THE APPRENTICESHIP OF HUMANISTIC CARING BY NURSE EDUCATORS: THE INFLUENCE OF NURSE EDUCATORS' LACK OF HUMANISTIC CARING ON STUDENTS' LEARNING

Dimitri Létourneau, PhD, RN

First and foremost, it is our belief that no educator makes the conscious choice of being "dehumanistic" toward students: It is rather a "sly and insidious" process, as described by Avoine (2012). Moreover, in agreement with Booth, Emerson, Hackney, and Souter (2016), we believe that clinical nursing and nursing education are two distinct disciplines and a "great nurse" is not necessarily a "great educator." However, as Roberts and Glod (2013) explained, some educators in the academic field may have less interest in education than they do in research activities. As a consequence, committing to students' success beyond what is generally required (i.e., the "extra steps") may seem less appealing for tenure purposes. If an educator does

not have genuine motivation and interest in being a caring educator, chances are that it will be visible in attitudes and behaviors. As
stated earlier in this book and as Mayeroff (1971/1990) pointed out,
Human Caring must be genuine; otherwise, it becomes a noncaring
obligation. It may, in other words, be perceived as "fake," and it may
impair both the students' and the educators' commitment to cocreate
a caring relationship.

In a phenomenological study conducted by Létourneau, Goudreau,
and Cara (2018) aiming at understanding the experience of learning to
care for the person with humanism, from the perspectives of nursing
students ($n = 18$) and nurses ($n = 8$), results shed some light on educators' dehumanizing practices and their potential impacts on learning.
Those practices had many forms, some being the educators' spoken
words and others being attitudes or behaviors.

Insufficient Acknowledgment of Students' Feelings and of Challenges in Their Learning

When it comes to spoken words, the results show that the "way"
things are said is sometimes more brutal than the content itself. For
instance, one second-year student, who we will call Hallay, recalled an
experience where she perceived harshness in the educator's response.
In short, this educator wanted to explain to students, who previously
shared their concerns about workload and academic results, that assessment was based on their assignments' performances and not on the
efforts put into them. Nevertheless, Hallay stated that this educator
told students "she wasn't there to assess efforts [they] put into [their]
work," which appears to be true, but was also perceived as devoid of
empathy in regard to their formerly shared concerns. If this educator had started by acknowledging and mentioning how hard it could
have been for students to complete their assignment, hopefully this
experience would not have been remembered as "negative" as it was.
Furthermore, if this educator had softened the way she explained how
assessment was preferred in this course (i.e., not based on efforts) and
showed openness and flexibility by asking students what their solutions to their concerns would have been, then again students could
have perceived that their concerns were really listened to. Hallay and
other participants mentioned that they felt an incongruence between
what they were asked to become (i.e., caring practitioners) with the
way they were "treated" as students. These participants identified

such incongruence as limiting their learning and feeding their cynicism. This cynicism consequently appeared to impede their interest in endorsing Human Caring for their future practice.

Lack of Interest in Students' Success and Learning

As for attitudes and behaviors, Shélanie, a third-year student, in her own words spoke about what Halldorsdottir (1991, 2013) calls the "life-neutral (biopassive) mode of being." Shélanie revealed that one of her educators, in contrast to others, did not appear interested in students' learning nor success. Instead, this educator was viewed as "someone who was giving assignments" rather than someone who embodied Human Caring in their way of being as a person. While this educator was not necessarily at the end of the "humanistic–dehumanistic" spectrum, it does look as if their attitudes did not make students feel that the educator was committed to helping the students become caring and humanistic nurses. Other participants encountered educators whose attitudes were described as "cold," "insensitive," or "detached" and this is closer to the "life-restraining (biostatic) mode of being" in Halldorsdottir's theory (1991, 2013). Because of these uncaring attitudes, Shélanie and other participants considered themselves less interested in acquiring knowledge from these educators: their passion for learning receded and their involvement in their courses declined.

Marked Hierarchical and Haughty Approach With Students

Some educators' approaches were perceived as hierarchical and haughty with students. Catherine, a second-year student, had clear memories of one faculty lecturer who made her, and her colleagues, feel belittled. In Catherine's own words, this faculty lecturer had a "superior look" on their face and seemed to be engaged in nursing education for reasons of prestige rather than for "good ones" (i.e., supporting students' learning). Catherine did not feel disrespected by this faculty lecturer; however, she did not believe that she could maintain a close student–educator relationship either. Additionally, she believed that this lecturer's approach was not congruent with Human Caring nor with humanism, which led Catherine to feel a greater distance between herself and the educator. As Catherine later added, "you appreciate that the people telling you to be humanistic embody humanism themselves," echoing Hallay's perceived incongruence.

Devaluation of Human Caring in the Clinical Setting

Clinical training is an area of nursing education that might be a little harder to inspire when it comes to caring practices. Even where a school's curriculum is to be grounded in Human Caring in agreement with Hills and Watson (2011), nurse preceptors (or clinical educators) in clinical settings might not believe in and encourage caring practices when accompanying students from said school. Indeed, we invite educators to remind themselves that despite all efforts put inside universities to promote a nursing practice anchored on Human Caring, clinical settings are imbued with a realistic aspect that is salient to students; hence, they represent what Duchscher (2001) called the "real world of nursing." That makes clinical training all the more important when it comes to ensuring humanistic approaches. Sadly, however, all too often, some nurse preceptors might undermine or undervalue Human Caring, sometimes implicitly and, at other times, explicitly. Shélanie later reflected on another lived experience where she felt that her nurse preceptor did not encourage nor view caring as a fundamental aspect of nursing. As Shélanie was trying to get to know her patient and when she later came back to her nurse preceptor to explain what she had learned from that patient, her nurse preceptor seemed uninterested and solely focused on medication to be soon administered. Shélanie added, "it was rather seen as a waste of time." Because nurse preceptors are responsible for students' assessment in their clinical training, giving rise to a power relationship as explained earlier in this chapter, certain students might make the choice of following what is asked by their nurse preceptor in order to obtain good grades, even though they are aware of an incongruence between what they are doing and what they wish to do (i.e., embody Human Caring). Not only does this prevent students from practicing and living caring in the moment, but it reinforces this idea of "theory–practice gap" between academic and clinical fields. For this reason, it is our belief that nurse educators also have the responsibility to inspire Human Caring in nurse preceptors.

The results from this phenomenological study appear to demonstrate that not only the theoretical content of Human Caring is important to students' learning but that it must be embodied by nurse educators in order to foster a caring praxis. We understand that not every faculty member might be passionate about nursing education, but we want to insist on their pivotal role in students' learning. As Catherine, a second-year student, recommended, it is to be humanistic to show [them] also how to be human-istic. In fact, everyone with everyone: the teachers, the tutors towards the students. It must be reciprocal, if the tutors and the professors display humanism, it might be easier for [them] to be humanistic because they are [their] role models after all. It's harder to manage, but nurse preceptors, without asking them to be "Godlike" humanists, but to encourage humanism. If it is espoused in the way of teaching, well it may be easier for [them] afterwards.

CONCLUSION

This chapter intended to raise nurse educators' consciousness about a darker aspect of nursing education: educators' dehumanizing practices toward students. After understanding this phenomenon and its impact on students and their learning, we discussed the importance of Human Caring to overcome the challenges in order to humanize nursing education, especially surrounding the student–educator relationships.

We have come to realize that, unfortunately, we are witnessing dehumanization in nursing education. Such dehumanization may have serious impacts on our students as well as their learning the profession. Létourneau's Pragmatic Segment exemplifies these impacts clearly. Moreover, Birks et al. (2014) argue that ineffectively controlling bullying problems in academia will have serious consequences for students as well as the nursing profession. How could we, as nurse educators, conquer these challenges and promote humanization in nursing education? We could teach with loving-kindness, act as role models for students, and promote a caring teaching/learning environment where students can feel safe to learn (Cara & Hills, 2018). We strongly believe that Human Caring will make a difference in our students' learning and lives, as it is our foremost responsibility.

The teacher's role is to nurture the learner: to nurture the ethical ideal, to nurture the caring role, to nurture the creative drive, to nurture curiosity and the search for satisfying ideas, to nurture assertiveness and the spirit of inquiry together with the desire to seek dialogue about care, and to be available for that dialogue. The teacher's role is to interact with students as persons of worth, dignity, intelligence, and high scholarly standards. (Bevis, 2000, p. 174)

REFERENCES

Adams, L. Y., & Maykut, C. (2015). Bullying: The antithesis of caring acknowledging the dark side of the nursing profession. *International Journal for Caring Sciences, 8*(3), 765–773. Retrieved from http://www.internationaljournalofcaringsciences .org/docs/28_Adams_special_8_3.pdf

Arslan, S., & Dinç, L. (2017). Nursing students' perceptions of faculty members' ethical/ unethical attitudes. *Nursing Ethics, 24*(7), 789–801. doi:10.1177/0969733015625366

Avoine, M.-P. (2012). *La signification de pratiques déshumanisantes telles que vécues par des patients hospitalisés ou ayant été hospitalisés en centre de réadaptation* (Master's thesis). Retrieved from ProQuest Dissertations & Theses. (UMI No. MR96229).

Avoine, M.-P., O'Reilly, L., & Michaud, C. (2012, May). *The signification of dehumanizing practices of nurses in a physical rehabilitation setting from the patient perspective: A phenomenological study.* Oral presentation at the 33rd Annual Conference, International Association for Human Caring, Philadelphia, PA.

Avoine, M.-P., O'Reilly, L., Michaud, C., & St-Cyr Tribble, D. (2011). Dehumanization in health care: A concept analysis. *International Journal for Human Caring, 15*(3), 60. doi:10.20467/1091-5710.15.3.59

Beck, C. T. (2001). Caring within nursing education: A metasynthesis. *Journal of Nursing Education, 40*(3), 101–109. doi:10.3928/0148-4834-20010301-04

Beck, D. M. (2015). Incivility and student and faculty relationships: Implications for revising mentorship programs for nurse educators. *SOJ Nursing & Health Care, 1*(1), 1–10. doi:10.15226/2471-6529/1/1/00103

Bevis, E. O. (2000). Teaching and learning: The key to education and professionalism. In E. O. Bevis & J. Watson (Eds.), *Toward a caring curriculum: A new pedagogy for nursing* (pp. 153–188). New York, NY: National League for Nursing.

Bevis, E. O., & Watson, J. (2000). *Toward a caring curriculum: A new pedagogy for nursing.* New York, NY: National League for Nursing. (Original work published 1989)

Birks, M., Budden, L. M., Stewart, L., & Chapman, Y. (2014). Editorial. Turning the tables: The growth of upward bullying in nursing academia. *Journal of Advanced Nursing, 70*(8), 1685–1687. doi:10.1179/pma.2014.48.1.001

Booth, T. L., Emerson, C. J., Hackney, M. G., & Souter, S. (2016). Preparation of academic nurse educators. *Nurse Education in Practice, 19*, 54–57. doi:10.1016/j .nepr.2016.04.006

Boykin, A., & Schoenhofer, S. O. (1993). *Nursing as caring: A model for transforming practice.* New York, NY: National League for Nursing.

Boykin, A., & Schoenhofer, S. O. (2001). *Nursing as caring: A model for transforming practice.* Sudbury, MA: Jones & Bartlett Publishers & National League for Nursing. (Original work published 1993)

Boykin, A., Touhy, T. A., & Smith, M. C. (2011). Evolution of a caring-based college of nursing. In M. Hills & J. Watson (Eds.), *Creating a Caring Science curriculum: An emancipatory pedagogy for nursing* (pp. 157–184). New York, NY: Springer Publishing Company.

Buber, M. (1996). *I and thou: A new translation, with a prologue and notes by Walter Kaufmann*. (W. Kaufmann, Trans.). New York, NY: Touchstone. (Original work published 1970)

Cara, C. (2017, June). *Rediscovering love, compassion, and caring to alleviate dehumanization*. Keynote speech presented at the 38th International Association for Human Caring Conference, Edmonton, AB, Canada.

Cara, C., Gauvin-Lepage, J., Lefebvre, H., Létourneau, D., Alderson, M., Larue, C., . . . Mathieu, C. (2016). Le Modèle humaniste des soins infirmiers—UdeM: Perspective novatrice et pragmatique. *Recherche en soins infirmiers, 125*, 20–31. doi:10.3917/rsi.125.0020

Cara, C., & Hills, M. (2018, May). *The added value of Caring Science: Its contributions to humanize nursing education*. Oral presentation at the Canadian Association of Schools in Nursing Conference, Montreal, QC, Canada.

Chan, Z. C., Tong, C. W., & Henderson, S. (2017). Power dynamics in the student-teacher relationship in clinical settings. *Nurse Education Today, 49*, 174–179. doi:10.1016/j.nedt.2016.11.026

Christoff, K. (2014). Dehumanization in organizational settings: Some scientific and ethical consideration. *Frontiers in Human Neuroscience, 8*(748), 1–5. doi:10.3389/fnhum.2014.00748

Duchscher, J. E. B. (2001). Out in the real world: Newly graduated nurses in acute-care speak out. *Journal of Nursing Administration, 31*, 426–439. Retrieved from http://journals.lww.com/jonajournal/Pages/default.aspx

Froneman, K., Du Plessis, E., & Koen, M. P. (2016). Effective educator–student relationships in nursing education to strengthen nursing students' resilience. *Curationis, 39*(1), 1595. doi:10.4102/curationis.v39i1.1595

Gillespie, M. (2005). Student–teacher connection: A place of possibility. *Journal of Advanced Nursing, 52*(2), 211–219. doi:10.1111/j.1365-2648.2005.03581.x

Halldorsdottir, S. (1990). The essential structure of a caring and uncaring encounter with a teacher: The perspective of the nursing student. In M. Leininger & J. Watson (Eds.), *The caring imperative in nursing education* (pp. 95–108). New York, NY: National League for Nursing Press.

Halldorsdottir, S. (1991). Five basic modes of being with another. In D. A. Gaut & M. Leininger (Eds.), *Caring: The compassionate* (pp. 37–49). New York, NY: National League for Nursing Press.

Halldorsdottir, S. (2013). Five basic modes of being with another. In M. C. Smith, M. C. Turkel, & Z. R. Wolf (Eds.), *Caring in nursing classics. An essential resource* (pp. 201–210). New York, NY: Springer Publishing Company.

Haslam, N. (2006). Dehumanization: An integrative review. *Personality and Social Psychology Review, 10*(3), 252–264. doi:10.1207/s15327957pspr1003_4

Hills, M., & Cara, C. (2019). Curriculum development processes and pedagogical practices for advancing Caring Science literacy. In W. Rosa, S. Horton-Deutsch, & J. Watson (Eds.), *A handbook for Caring Science: Expanding the paradigm* (pp. 197–210). New York, NY: Springer Publishing Company.

Hills, M., & Watson, J. (2011). *Creating a Caring Science curriculum: An emancipatory pedagogy for nursing*. New York, NY: Springer Publishing Company.

Labrague, L. J., McEnroe-Petitte, D. M., Papathanasiou, I. V., Edet, O. B., & Arulappan, J. (2015). Impact of instructors' caring on students' perceptions of their own caring behaviors: Students' caring. *Journal of Nursing Scholarship, 47*(4), 338–346. doi:10.1111/jnu.12139

Létourneau, D., Cara, C., & Goudreau, J. (2017). Humanizing nursing care: An analysis of caring theories through the lens of humanism. *International Journal for Human Caring, 21*(1), 32–40. doi:10.20467/1091-5710-21.1.32

Létourneau, D., Goudreau, J., & Cara, C. (2018, May). *The experience of learning to care for the person with humanism: A phenomenological study*. Communication presented at the 39th Annual International Association for Human Caring Conference, Minneapolis, MN.

Mayeroff, M. (1990). *On caring*. New York, NY: Harper Perennial. (Original work published 1971)

Miller, B. K., Haber, J., & Byrne, N. W. (1990). The experience of caring in the teaching process of nursing education: Student and teacher perspectives. In M. M. Leininger & J. Watson (Eds.), *The caring imperative in education* (pp. 255–266). New York, NY: National League for Nursing Press.

Muliira, J. K., Natarajan, J., & van der Colff, J. (2017). Nursing faculty academic incivility: Perceptions of nursing students and faculty. *BMC Medical Education, 17*(1), 1–10. doi:10.1186/s12909-017-1096-8

National League for Nursing. (1988). *Curriculum revolution: Mandate for change*. New York, NY: National League for Nursing Press.

National League for Nursing. (2003). *Position statement. Innovation in nursing education: A call to reform*. Retrieved from http://www.nln.org/docs/default-source/about/archived-position-statements/innovation-in-nursing-education-a-call-to-reform-pdf.pdf

Noddings, N. (2013). *Caring. A relational approach to ethics and moral education*. Berkeley: University of California Press.

Reason, P. (Ed.). (1994). *Participation in human inquiry*. London, UK: Sage.

Roach, M. S. (1984). *Caring: The human mode of being, implications for nursing*. Toronto, ON, Canada: University of Toronto.

Roach, M. S. (2002). *Caring, the human mode of being: A blueprint for the health professions* (2nd ed.). Ottawa, ON, Canada: Cambridge Health Alliance Press.

Roberts, S. J., & Glod, C. (2013). Faculty roles: Dilemmas for the future of nursing education. *Nursing Forum, 48*, 99–105. doi:10.1111/nuf.12018

Rogers, C. R. (1961). *On becoming a person: A therapist's view of psychotherapy*. Boston, MA: Houghton Mifflin Company.

Seibel, L. M., & Fehr, F. C. (2018). "They can crush you": Nursing students' experiences of bullying and the role of faculty. *Journal of Nursing Education and Practice, 8*(6), 66–76. doi:10.5430/jnep.v8n6p66

Smith, Y. M., & Crowe, A. R. (2017). Nurse educator perceptions of the importance of relationship in online teaching and learning. *Journal of Professional Nursing, 33*(1), 11–19. doi:10.1016/j.profnurs.2016.06.004

Stagg, S. J., Sheridan, D. J., Jones, R. A., & Speroni, K. G. (2013). Workplace bullying: The effectiveness of a workplace program. A systematic review. *Workplace Health and Safety, 61*(8), 333–338. doi:10.1177/216507991306100803

Thomas, C. M. (2010). Teaching nursing students and newly registered nurses strategies to deal with violent behaviors in the professional practice environment. *Journal of Continuing Education in Nursing, 41*(7), 299–310. doi:10.3928/00220124-20100401-09

Watson, J. (1988). *Nursing: Human science and human care* (2nd ed.). New York, NY: National League for Nursing. (Original work published 1985)

Watson, J. (2008). *Nursing: The philosophy and science of caring* (revised ed.). Boulder: University Press of Colorado.

Watson, J. (2012). *Human Caring Science: A theory of nursing* (2nd ed.). Sudbury, MA: Jones & Bartlett Learning.

Whealan, J. (2017). The Caring Science imperative: A hallmark in nursing education. In S. Lee, P. Palmieri, & J. Watson (Eds.), *Global advances in Human Caring literacy* (pp. 33–42). New York, NY: Springer Publishing Company.

Zander, R. S., & Zander, B. (2002). *The art of possibility.* New York, NY: Penguin Group.

Ziefle, K. (2018). Incivility in nursing education: Generational differences. *Teaching and Learning in Nursing, 13*(1), 27–30. doi:10.1016/j.teln.2017.09.004

2

Educators' Caring Values, Attitudes, and Behaviors That Contribute to the Humanization of Nursing Education

Becoming aware of your beliefs and assumptions, particularly in relation to how they "show up" in your behavior, can prove to be a very insightful exercise. Many of us behave without really being aware of what is driving our behavior, not being aware of how we "see the world" through our own value lens.
—Hills and Watson, 2011, p. 31

LEARNING INTENTIONS

- Reflect how Human Caring values may inform nurse educators to be and become caring teachers.
- Explore how adopting various caring attitudes in teaching practice may assist nurse educators to recognize students as unique human beings.
- Appreciate how caring behaviors can promote students' learning.

- Understand how Human Caring values, attitudes, and behaviors may support nurse educators' moral imperative to humanize nursing education.
- Learn concrete strategies to promote Human Caring values, attitudes, and behaviors in nursing education.

INTRODUCTION

This chapter guides nurse educators on how to use Human Caring values, attitudes, and behaviors in their efforts to humanize nursing education. After introducing Human Caring in general, we present essential Human Caring values, attitudes, and behaviors of nurse educators and discuss how they contribute to promoting students' learning. We conclude with a Pragmatic Segment that also helps to illustrate and differentiate between caring values, attitudes, and behaviors in nursing education.

HUMAN CARING IN NURSING EDUCATION
Relevance of Human Caring in Nursing Education

Nursing literature has demonstrated the significance of Human Caring mainly within the clinical domain (Boykin & Schoenhofer, 2013; Duffy, 2018; Lee, Palmieri, & Watson, 2017; Rosa, Horton-Deutsch, & Watson, 2019; Smith, Turkel, & Wolf, 2013; Swanson, 2013; Watson, 2008, 2012). However, a caring perspective is relevant not just to nurses' clinical practice. Caring can also inspire nurse educators to facilitate their students' awareness, consciousness, and learning in order for them to develop caring relationships with their patients and to become caring nurses. Indeed, a caring perspective can prompt nurse educators to consider students as coparticipants or contributors, thus inviting a cocreation of knowledge relevant for their future caring practice. This contribution of Human Caring to nursing education has recently become more recognized in the nursing education literature (Beck, 2001; Bevis & Watson, 2000; Hills & Cara, 2019; Hills & Watson, 2011; Touhy & Boykin, 2008).

But what is Human Caring and how can nurse educators be informed by it in their daily practice of nursing education?

Human Caring: The Metaphor of the Iceberg

We define Human Caring in nursing education as *a relational and humanistic way to teach and develop a caring relationship with students in order to promote*

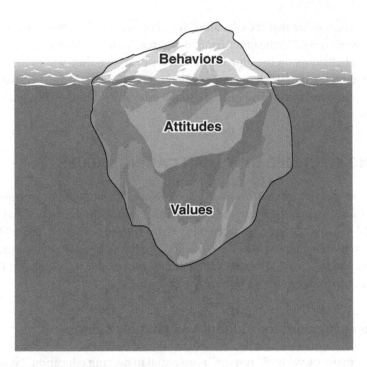

Figure 2.1 Caring: The metaphor of the iceberg.

learning and meaning while preserving dignity. Learning occurs within the nurse educator–student relationship, guiding students to new meaning and knowledge integration as well as an expanded consciousness in regard to one's own caring–healing praxis.

We use the metaphor of an iceberg to explain Human Caring (Cara, 2004, 2017). Human Caring is composed of behaviors, values, and attitudes but, as with an iceberg, much of what constitutes Human Caring is not readily apparent (see Figure 2.1). One can see only a part of Human Caring, caring behaviors, whereas values and attitudes lie beneath.

Behaviors are our observable actions; unlike values or attitudes, they can be measured. *Values* are engrained and deep-rooted elements that one "gives worth to" and by which one wants to live one's personal and professional life. *Attitudes* are psychological dispositions that guide one's behaviors. Human Caring originates from humanist values, influencing our attitudes, which guide our behaviors.

Values are of foremost importance; they provide stability to the Human Caring iceberg. For example, if you teach nurse educators to adopt certain behaviors, such as greeting students with a smile in front of the classroom or giving them positive feedback, without linking these behaviors to humanistic values, chances are that the educators' usual behaviors will return in a period of crisis or stress. On the other hand, if you teach nurse educators to ground learned behaviors on the humanistic value of respect, they will more likely understand the importance of those behaviors in order to show their respect to students, and in a period of crisis, nurse educators' humanistic behaviors will prevail.

BEING INFORMED BY HUMAN CARING VALUES

We now discuss what it means to use Human Caring values in nursing education. As previously stated, we define "values" as elements that are judged worthwhile and that guide one's attitudes and behaviors. We explore respect, human dignity, belief in students' potential, freedom of choice and action, and integrity. We give examples, and nurse educators will also have the opportunity to explore other caring values.

Valuing Respect for Students as Human Beings

The humanistic value of "respect" is essential in nursing education. Numerous authors consider it to be of utmost importance in the clinical domain (Boykin & Schoenhofer, 1993/2001; Cara, 2004, 2017; Cara et al., 2016; Lazenby, 2017; O'Reilly, Cara, & Delmas, 2016; Ray, 2010; Roach, 2002; Swanson, 2013; Watson, 2012, 2018). As it is crucial to patient care, respect is also recognized as an essential value within nursing education. But, in this context, what does respect mean exactly (Beck, 2001; Bevis & Watson, 2000; Boykin, 1994; Cara & Hills, 2018; Hills & Cara, 2019; Hills & Watson, 2011)?

To respect someone (e.g., a student or a colleague) is to show unconditional positive regard to the person simply because the person is a human being. We define respect as displaying the highest regard and reverence for all human beings, knowing that respect is the keystone to any relationship. In the domain of nursing education, to respect students is to honor them as unique and whole individuals, aspiring to become caring nurses.

As an example, nurse educators would ground their behaviors on respect for their students by answering their questions in a timely manner. Or nurse educators would express admiration for graduate students sharing divergent ideas, acknowledge the significance of their work, and encourage them to publish it in a journal. By embracing respect, nurse educators have their students' best interest at heart and perceive their role as guide, facilitator, or mentor.

Respect is fundamental to learning. At this point, it is relevant to explain our perspective on students' learning, as it is not simply an outcome to be categorized, evaluated, and graded at the end of a class. Rather, learning is a process wherein students must understand, reflect, and develop new knowledge in order for them to grasp and appreciate their future caring practice. Accordingly, providing a learning environment filled with respect will help students to feel comfortable sharing their experiences and learning new knowledge. Nurse educators could humanize nursing education by, for example, respecting students' individual and unique learning rhythms and by honoring their future contributions to the nursing discipline and profession. Being grounded in this humanistic value, nurse educators would perceive their role as creating a caring–trusting teaching/learning environment. This environment, in which respect for students is always demonstrated, can assist them in learning at a higher and deeper consciousness regarding one's own future caring praxis.

Valuing Students' Human Dignity

The second humanistic value concerns "human dignity." It is frequently linked, in the nursing literature, to the value of respect. As Roach (2002) explains, caring implies to reflect "on what it means to be a human person, and on the canons of respect for human dignity which are the guardians of both personhood and community" (p. 3).

In the clinical arena, several authors have discussed human dignity as being essential to Human Caring (Cara et al., 2016; Ray, 2010; Roach, 2002; Swanson, 2013; Watson, 2008, 2012, 2018). According to Watson (2012), it is the nurses' moral ideal or imperative to preserve people's human dignity. To our knowledge, in nursing education, human dignity has rarely been considered paramount and is often used interchangeably with the word "respect." But how is it important in nursing education?

To preserve a person's human dignity in nursing education means to consider students as unique and whole individuals, never objectifying them, nor perceiving or treating them as objects, or violating their rights. Being inspired by this value, nurse educators would consider students as active whole human beings contributing to their own learning, rather than objectifying them as passive objects only receiving or accumulating information, which may impair their personhood. Sadly, we often realize the importance of human dignity after it is lost, for example, treating a student as an object—"the tall French redhead student in the last row"—or insinuating that a particular student's question is insignificant or irrelevant.

Similarly, in the classroom, students may also experience a lack of human dignity in different ways, for example:

- Feeling humiliated during laboratory practices
- Being stigmatized or labeled as a "weak student"
- Being considered stupid as a result of questions asked in class
- Being considered too slow during procedural techniques training
- Not being able to participate in the decision regarding a class assignment
- Having the nurse educator disclose the student's failure in front of others
- Perceiving racial or gender discrimination in the classroom

Nurse educators have a responsibility not to ignore such dehumanizing students' experiences revealing a reduced human dignity, but instead to become a strong students' advocate. As Bevis (2000) states,

> teachers of nurses have a special responsibility as do nurses who practice in settings where students learn. These nurses can be instrumental in being the students' mirror, revealing to the students things about themselves that will nurture the ethical ideal or destroy it. (p. 184)

Nurse educators can embody their valuing of human dignity in their classrooms by suggesting that everyone be open to each other's uniqueness and diversity in order for students to learn in a "humanistic space." Hills and Watson (2011) use the term "safe space" when considering students' vulnerability and discovery of personal meaning. It is critical for students to learn in safety so that they can explore delicate or controversial issues. A Human Caring perspective "seeks to preserve human dignity and honor the whole person for learning *and* healing; it is open to inner exploration for meaning and personal knowing, and, thus, the transformation and evolution of human consciousness" (Hills & Watson, 2011, p. 36). Maintaining their human dignity will support and nurture students' growth and emancipation. Such a perspective can only contribute to humanizing nursing education.

Valuing and Believing in Students' Potential

The third humanistic value, which we perceive to be important, is "believing in the students' potential." This value has not been discussed as intensively as the previous two, even in the clinical domain. Nevertheless, we believe it to be crucial, especially in nursing education.

Such a value invites nurse educators to believe in their students' potential to learn, grow, and succeed as future professional caring nurses. As caring nurse educators, we need to have confidence that our students are able to acquire knowledge, skills, and competence in the discipline. If you do not believe that they are able to learn, you might not accompany them in their learning process and recognize their abilities to learn to become caring nurses. Nurse educators informed by this value will not lose faith or give up on their students. They will not abandon the idea that they can succeed. Instead of anticipating certain students' failure in class, caring nurse educators would see their role as facilitating, supporting, and accompanying these students in their learning process. Such educators would assist students to appreciate their own strengths and help them find useful resources to complete their program with accomplishment.

Mayeroff (1971), an important humanist philosopher, refers to the "potential for growth" in several of his "caring ingredients." For example, "patience," "trust," and "hope" enable others to grow in their own time and own way through caring (Mayeroff, 1971). More specifically to the education domain, Mayeroff explains that to promote students' growth, you must consider them as the center of your attention.

In other words, nurse educators embodying this value in their classrooms will consider students' learning as central and trust that they can succeed with proper guidance and support. Of course, students must also invest in their learning. This perspective is fundamental to humanizing nursing education.

Valuing Students' Freedom of Choice and Action

The fourth humanistic value that we view as relevant in nursing education is acknowledging "students' freedom of choice and action."

In nursing education, it is important to acknowledge that students always have a choice about the meaning they attribute to their learning. Hence, nurse educators informed by this value will be more likely to adopt nonpaternalistic pedagogical approaches in order to promote students' freedom of choice, autonomy, and inner wisdom. A concrete example would be to involve students in participating in some decision-making in the classroom regarding, for example, the class assignment format (e.g., oral presentation, roundtable of dialogue and discourse, paper for future publication). Fostering the students' autonomy suggests encouraging them to develop an active learning process instead of a passive approach to obtain knowledge. In doing so, nurse educators will also recognize students' liberty to reflect and learn as they desire, by encouraging their creativity in regard to their novice caring–healing praxis. Similarly, this honors the student's individual search for personal meaning and inner wisdom, which almost always goes beyond what is written in textbooks. Such a viewpoint subscribes to humanizing nursing education.

Watson proposes a nursing education approach

> freeing human potential, an approach that allows one to develop not only rational and moral capacities, but emotional, expressive, intuitive, esthetic, personal capacities and bring one's full self to bear with one's life work—in this instance, work of human caring. Changes in nursing education and practice can anticipate the highest development of a person as one engaged and committed to human caring as a way of being—as person and as professional with equal privileges and opportunities to study and practice one's life work. (Bevis & Watson, 2000, p. 47)

This value is also coherent with Hills and Watson's (2011) work on emancipatory pedagogy. In that context, believing in students' freedom of choice implies encouraging a relationship between the nurse educator, the student, and the knowledge, the latter being linked to the student's lived experiences and meanings. In other words, for students to reach transformative learning, nurse educators shall encourage them to reflect on a real nursing situation, lived in their respective recent clinical practice, in order to attempt to find their own meaning within this caring experience.

Valuing Global Integrity

The fifth and final relevant humanistic value is "global integrity." In the domain of nursing education, this last value invites nurse educators to become role models for students, accompanying students as they learn about the importance of honesty, accountability, and imputability in the nursing profession. Both nurse educators and school administrators must cocreate a culture of professional integrity, evident throughout the school, whether in the classroom or in clinical practice settings, for all people, that is, students, educators, administrators, and other workers.

In their concept analysis of integrity, Devine and Chin (2018) claim that it has been considered, in the nursing literature, mostly in association with nurses' or students' professional conduct in both clinical practice and education. They argue that the concept of "integrity" has often been discussed as a "lack of integrity," corresponding, for example, to cheating, plagiarism, and falsifying documentations. With the expansion of plagiarism in schools, this value is therefore of great importance in nursing education.

Nurse educators can assist students to understand the meaning of integrity as it pertains to their actual role as nursing students and also their future role as professionals. For example, nurse educators can embody this value in their clinical supervision by encouraging students to achieve reflective practice in order to provide the best care possible to their patients. Reflective practice is essential to nurse educators themselves and also to teach students about advanced nursing practice, clinical leadership, and social actions, all of which can contribute to their reflection about nursing's larger social mission.

TIME OUT FOR REFLECTION

Write your reflection in a journal in order to link the preceding theoretical segment with your personal teaching/learning experiences.

Think about your personal teaching/learning experiences, and then ask yourself the following questions:

- How well have these preceding values fit with your current teaching/learning practice?
- Which ones are the most important for you?
- From your perceptions, what are the impacts of these values for your students?
- Are there other humanistic values that are important for you?
- What are some strategies that you can implement to ground, even more, your teaching/learning practice in humanistic values?

EXAMPLES OF NURSE EDUCATORS' CARING ATTITUDES

As mentioned earlier, "attitudes" are psychological dispositions that guide one's own behaviors. One can inquire about nurse educators' essential caring attitudes relevant to humanize nursing education.

Examples of nurse educators' caring attitudes with their students include the following:

- Showing compassion toward students experiencing failure
- Having an interest in students' lived experiences and meanings
- Being present to students in their learning process
- Being committed to assist students in their learning
- Wanting to understand through openness students' lived experiences

We give examples, and nurse educators will also have the possibility to explore other caring attitudes that might be expressing a humanistic teaching/learning practice.

Compassion Toward Students

We believe that "compassion toward students" is an important caring attitude in nursing education. It represents nurse educators acknowledging students' distress, trying to understand their lived experience, and seeking solutions to relieve their distress in some way.

For example, nurse educators may have compassion for students who have been experiencing serious learning challenges in class or in the nursing program. Compassionate nurse educators would first acknowledge their distress regarding their probable failure and then communicate support and clarification in order for students to grasp the important learning in class. Moreover, by attempting to transform a negative experience into a positive learning experience, nurse educators can incorporate compassion as part of their caring teaching/learning praxis.

According to Roach (2002), "compassion" is an attribute of caring, one of her 6Cs. She explains compassion as sharing the pain and suffering of a person, in our case students, and being changed by such experience. Vachon (2019), an expert psychologist on compassion, defines it as

> noticing or recognizing suffering, being empathically resonant with that person, desiring to relieve that suffering, and acting to attempt to alleviate that suffering in some way. . . . This compassion, however, should not be viewed as simply an emotional response or just good communication skills . . . compassion is a motivational process that generates a particular pattern in the brain that aligns our attention, cognition, and emotions in a compassionate response to [students]. It is the focused channeling of our competence in response to [students'] suffering, not simply empathic resonation and expressing concern. (p. 64)

Moreover, van der Cingel (2014) speaks of seven dimensions of compassion: "attentiveness," "active listening," "naming of suffering," "involvement," "helping," "being present," and "understanding" (p. 1255). These dimensions of compassion may be useful to nurse educators in order to display such an attitude with students who are failing. Consider, as an example, a third-year female student who is struggling in her clinical practice course. The nurse educator could manifest compassion by expressing "attentiveness," showing an interest in the student's lived experience as a human being. From the nurse educator's "active listening," the caring nurse educator can invite the student to share her story, revealing emotions such as anger, loss, and despair. By acknowledging the distress and difficulties within the student's experience, the nurse educator is "naming the suffering." To acknowledge suffering is relevant "because it turns suffering into a visible aspect of life, instead of something that one should keep to oneself" (van der Cingel, 2014, p. 1255). By accompanying the student through the expression of emotions and distress in a safe environment, the caring nurse educator exhibits "involvement." Subsequently, by "helping" the student to assess her needs and to find solutions, for example, by asking the dean for the evaluation to be revised or by taking the clinical practice course again next year, the nurse educator is actually "acting to attempt to alleviate that suffering in some way" (Vachon, 2019, p. 64). By "being there," the nurse educator conveys that the student is important as a human being. Lastly, when the caring nurse educator expresses understanding of the student's lived experience of failure, charged with distress, loss, despair, and suffering, they are able to communicate compassion, which represents "a moral answer to suffering" (van der Cingel, 2014, p. 1257).

Presence in Students' Learning Process

We believe that "presence in students' learning process" is an important caring attitude in nursing education. In fact, nurse educators' presence is critical to students' learning.

For example, in an undergraduate class during a group discussion, when a student tentatively asks a question, a caring nurse educator would be present to that student by moving closer to the student, making eye contact, and responding in a way that demonstrates openness, empathy, and respect, even if the question may appear to be less relevant.

Another example is when working with a graduate student who is feeling low self-esteem and lacks confidence as they are about to deliver an oral presentation to a large scholarly conference. By "being there" and "being with" the student in a profound caring relationship, the nurse educator can listen to the student's anxiety and fear, remain positive and supportive in order to find solutions, and foster confidence and well-being, to eventually be able to deliver the oral presentation with assurance. The nurse educator would need to stay in the student's frame of reference, without being judgmental. It is the nurse educator's presence and caring consciousness, within the caring moment with the student, that would allow the nurse educator to open their heart and mind to the lived experience of the student. The nurse educator being fully present would give the student time and space to progress and transform. Through presence, the caring nurse educator can nurture the student's learning process and personhood.

Different types of presence are discussed in the literature. Nurse educators' presence requires an awareness beyond a physical presence. As Watson (2018) explains, "authentic presence in a given moment between [a nurse educator and a student] captures the human-to-human, spirit-to-spirit connection, which is felt experientially but may not be detected by an outside objective observer" (p. 90). In other terms, students in need may sense the authentic presence of nurse educators while other students or colleagues might not.

In her concept analysis, Boeck (2014) talks about "genuine presence." She proclaims that "genuine nursing presence" corresponds to being with another person, deeply listening, and not being centered on one's own intervention but rather being present within the intimacy of the moment. "Genuinely present" nurse educators would be open and embracing students in their journey and would provide support, comfort, and reassurance to their students.

Commitment to Students' Learning Journey

Nurse educators' "commitment to students' learning journey" of the discipline of nursing, or "nursology" (Fawcett & Chinn, 2019), is another pivotal caring attitude. This attitude is linked to nurse educators' moral sense of duty. A Human Caring perspective guides nurse educators to a moral commitment to protect students' human dignity. Being committed, as nurse educators, conveys a real consciousness of being present with loving-kindness and compassion for students, as unique individuals, as well as to their learning and success. Hence, nurse educators' commitment is central in displaying humanization in nursing education.

Nurse educators demonstrating their responsibility, imputability, and enthusiasm toward students' learning and successful accomplishment in their classrooms as well as their overall academic success in the nursing program would convey their commitment not only to students but also to their school and nursing education. Consequently, nurse educators' commitment comes across as being linked to their moral imperative to act according to an ethic of caring.

For Roach (2002), "commitment" corresponds to an attribute of caring, another of her 6Cs. She explains that commitment is important for professionals in terms of accountability and responsibility. She defines commitment as "a complex affective response characterized by a convergence between one's desires and one's obligations, and by a deliberate choice to act in accordance with them" (p. 62). She insists that a nurse's commitment should extend far beyond a preference or willingness to respond. Commitment could be seen as related to nurse educators' firm choice of investing themselves, which is internalized as an obligation yet never to be considered as a burden. In that sense, nurse educators' commitment to students' learning journey could be linked to an ethic of caring that involves a commitment to people.

Halldorsdottir's (1990) seminal work also identified "commitment" as an important aspect of teaching. In her phenomenological study aimed to understand caring and uncaring encounters with a teacher, from the perspective of nine nursing students in Iceland, she identified "professional commitment" as a theme. "This important quality of professional caring is evidenced by the teacher's enthusiasm for own subject, sense of vision, high regard for nurses and nursing, professional activity, and search for excellence" (p. 99).

Promoting Mutual Trust Within Nurse Educator–Student Relationships

Mutual trust within the nurse educator–student relationship is another caring attitude in nursing education that we consider fundamental.

Mutual trust is acknowledging each other's uniqueness as human beings and knowing that each person is reliable, dependable, and responsible. This involves having confidence to share and communicate honestly. Therefore, within caring teaching/learning relationships, both mutuality and trust are central to have each other's respect, where both educators and students are valued and of equal importance.

For example, nurse educators wanting to establish a caring relationship with new graduate students may want to create a sense of mutual trust at the beginning. In so doing, nurse educators will help students realize that their teacher will be there for them during the entire graduate nursing program, all the way until completion. Students will then feel free and safe to ask questions and discuss their anxiety, fears, and preoccupations regarding the upcoming project. Consequently, this caring attitude helps nurse educators to humanize nursing education.

In fact, Halldorsdottir's (1990) research findings reveal that students' perspectives of caring encounters with a teacher include "mutual trust" as an important cornerstone of student–teacher working relationships. She explains that

> it also involves mutual communication of acceptance, as well as mutual acknowledgement of each other's uniqueness as persons. Successful completion of this phase establishes the bond between the teacher and the student . . . where the student feels safe enough to open up and

speak the truth to the teacher . . . and trusts the teacher to be truthful in giving honest feedback. (p. 100)

Moreover, mutual trust promotes learning, growth, and emancipation for both students and nurse educators. Indeed, mutual trust between nurse educators and students can assist students in learning its importance for their future relationships with patients and families. Therefore, nurse educators, establishing a mutual trusting relationship with students, demonstrates how students can *be* and *become* caring nurses with their patients, families, and communities. Mutual trust can also help nurse educators find meaning in their daily caring teaching/learning praxis by recognizing that they make a difference in their students' lives and learning processes.

TIME OUT FOR REFLECTION

We invite you to write your reflection in a journal in order to link the preceding theoretical segment with your personal teaching/learning experiences.

Think about your personal teaching/learning experiences, and then ask yourself the following questions:

- How well do these preceding caring attitudes fit with your current teaching/learning practice?
- Which ones are the most important for you?
- Which ones are the most important to enhance caring relationships with your students?
- From your experiences, how do these caring attitudes contribute to your students' learning and success?
- Are there other caring attitudes that are important for you?

EXAMPLES OF NURSE EDUCATORS' CARING BEHAVIORS

Lastly, we present some examples of important nurse educators' caring behaviors that are possible to observe. Moreover, nurse educators will also have the possibility to explore other caring behaviors that might contribute to humanize nursing education. Table 2.1 outlines some examples of nurse educators' caring behaviors with their students and how they are linked to the preceding caring values. Hills and Watson (2011) explain that values

Table 2.1 Examples of Educators' Caring Behaviors and Their Links to Caring Values

Educators' Caring Behaviors	Links With Caring Values
Greet students in the classroom	Demonstrates your respect toward students
Consider students as unique individuals	Demonstrates your respect toward students
Provide availability to answer students' questions	Demonstrates your respect toward students
Encourage dialogue and discussion with students rather than lecturing to them	Demonstrates that you are valuing students' freedom of choice from an emancipatory pedagogy perspective
Recognize students' efforts in their assignments	Demonstrates that you are valuing and believing in students' potential
Provide positive feedback, support, and guidance to students	Demonstrates that you are valuing and believing in students' potential
Create a classroom environment committed to openness, where students feel safe to share their feelings and perspectives	Demonstrates your respect toward students and their human dignity Demonstrates that you are valuing students' freedom of choice from an emancipatory pedagogy perspective
Encourage each student to participate in the classroom discussion	Demonstrates that you are valuing and believing in students' potential Demonstrates that you are valuing students' freedom of choice from an emancipatory pedagogy perspective
Accompany students to find personal meaning in their learning experiences	Demonstrates that you value students' freedom of choice and their human dignity from an emancipatory pedagogy perspective
Listen to preoccupations identified by students and suggest strategies to solve issues	Demonstrates your respect toward students Demonstrates your global integrity
Encourage students to keep hope in regard to their academic success	Demonstrates that you are valuing students' human dignity and believing in students' potential

(continued)

Table 2.1 **Examples of Educators' Caring Behaviors and Their Links to Caring Values** *(Continued)*

Educators' Caring Behaviors	Links With Caring Values
Acknowledge students' learning in their class project	Demonstrates that you are valuing and believing in students' potential
Encourage students' critique of knowledge and be open to multiple truths	Demonstrates that you are valuing students' freedom of choice from an emancipatory pedagogy perspective
Celebrate students' success in the classroom	Demonstrates that you are valuing and believing in students' potential

are reflected in nurse educators' behaviors. In other words, several of these behaviors can contribute to humanize nursing education.

This list is not meant to be exhaustive, but it is intended to give some concrete examples to assist you in identifying your own caring behaviors and their related values.

TIME OUT FOR REFLECTION

We invite you to write your reflection in a journal in order to link the preceding theoretical segment with your personal teaching/learning experiences.

Think about your personal teaching/learning experiences, and then ask yourself the following questions:

- How well do the caring behaviors discussed fit with your current teaching/learning practice?
- Which ones are the most important for you?
- Which ones are the most important to enhance caring relationships with your students?
- Which ones are the most important to enhance students' learning?
- For each of the caring behaviors and values outlined earlier, think of one impact for each that students may experience.
- Are there other caring behaviors that are important for you or for your students?

PRAGMATIC SEGMENT
EXEMPLARS OF NURSE EDUCATORS' HUMAN CARING VALUES, ATTITUDES, AND BEHAVIORS

Zane Robinson Wolf, PhD, RN, CNE, FAAN

Students admitted to nursing programs attend physical and virtual campuses in the hope of a personal transformation: as baccalaureate-degree graduates who in turn pass the professional nurse-licensing exams; as graduate students seeking advanced degrees as clinicians, administrators, and educators; and as doctoral students aiming to expand their expertise for clinical, teaching, and research careers. Faculty and administrators of nursing programs respond to students' aspirations by offering the best curricula possible.

Beyond the Formal Curriculum
Over the course of a given program of studies, faculty members carry out formal, cocurricular, and hidden (Chen, 2015) curricula. The formal curriculum, reviewed and approved by nurse education accrediting bodies, is often visible in published programs of study that are consistent with a mission and structured by program goals and outcome statements and student learning outcomes for courses. Examples consist of didactic and clinical courses and simulations experienced by undergraduate and graduate students and delivered by faculty members and program administrators. Cocurricular activities, expressions of another curriculum, function outside of the formal, conventional curriculum (Chan, Liu, Fung, Tsang, & Yuen, 2018). Faculty members and students welcome cocurricular experiences because they help to expand students' awareness and development, for example, through service learning trips at home and internationally. They also include attendance at professional meetings, such as Sigma Theta Tau International chapter meetings, student association meetings, and professional organization meetings created for nursing specialty practice roles. Lastly, many examples of nursing's hidden curriculum are found in clinical practice settings. Students confront the conflicts in clinical practice settings and the ideals espoused in the formal curriculum, such as insufficient time available for staff nurses to develop caring relationships with patients.

Nurse Educators' Human Caring Values, Attitudes, and Behaviors
Throughout the educational process, faculty members witness students' vulnerability and at the same time convey the standards and the cultural norms, values, attitudes, and behaviors of nursing. Many examples of their caring work, from my long history as nursing faculty member and dean, are lived daily by the teachers and administrators of professional nursing as students build competencies and expertise.

Belief in Students' Potential
Faculty members are inspired as new students arrive with each academic year and semester; faculty members believe in students' great potential, an essential caring value, as a teacher. A nurse educator's faith is confirmed as students engage in and succeed throughout the many steps in theory and clinical courses and in cocurricular activities. One exemplar is seen in the great belief of a faculty member in undergraduate students. This faculty member doggedly coaches students who are challenged by test anxiety and/or knowledge deficits in anticipation of taking the professional nurse-licensing exam. This faculty member is consistently available to senior students and has created and modified a success program, consistent with the program's overall initiative for all student levels. This faculty member teaches content along with other faculty members, separate from and cocurricular with scheduled courses of the formal curriculum. This faculty member helps students visualize handling the testing situation, decipher the structure of test questions, and manage their disappointments as predictor test scores fall short. This faculty member teaches students to persist in their preparation efforts while demonstrating persistence with and belief in them. This faculty member never stops supporting students and celebrates points of intermediate and final success.

Another example of a faculty member's belief in students follows. A graduate nursing student for whom English is her second language apologized to her faculty. The student called herself a "senior" nurse who should have, from her perspective, known punctuation and grammar details in a paper. Her draft paper was excellent in content, organization, flow, and citations. The faculty member praised the student; the faculty member saw the student's present ability and her potential in writing an outstanding research proposal. The faculty member gently cautioned the student not to fault her efforts.

Respect for Students

Additionally, administrators also show their respect for students, a significant caring value in nursing education. For example, a dean of nursing education created an undergraduate nursing student advisory committee as a formal structure in the school, which provided an opportunity for students to bring complaints and concerns to the table. This committee consisted of students enrolled in different levels of the curriculum, a faculty chairperson, and the undergraduate director. At the time, the rigors of the curriculum were especially acute for the prelicensure students. Topics presented by students included personal safety concerns on campus, complaints about clinical placements that taxed students' transportation reserves, and the need for more flexible schedules in the simulation lab. By listening to and acting to resolve some issues, the dean and undergraduate chair showed respect for students' experiences. Simultaneously, the administrators served as role models for comportment during meetings and for ways to mediate conflicts. The committee still functions today.

Knowing Students as Unique Individuals

When considering student enrollment counts for in-person classes, clinical settings, and simulation laboratory experiences and the virtual environments of online courses, nurse faculty are tasked with learning about the uniqueness of each student. Faculty members' exemplars are many. Efforts to know students as individuals have involved mapping a classroom's seating locations to learn students' names, seeing students' interactivity during class sessions, and more. Another exemplar is seen in a discussion option in a learning management system. When used in both face-to-face or online-only teaching, students are provided an opportunity to connect and are invited to match a faculty member's introduction by sharing details about themselves. Also, students are encouraged to use threading discussions, student-to-student. One faculty member goes beyond this strategy during phone calls by asking about graduate and doctoral students' workplaces and roles, names of basic nursing education programs, family composition, and other details as they provide critique, offer advice, and share next steps in the course and its assignments. Students know how to contact the faculty member and what times are good for phone conversations. The faculty member encourages students to email, yet states a preference for phone contact and provides them with a cell phone number. Even though student–faculty relationships may be brief, and despite being constrained by each week's responsibilities and timeline of a course, they often represent meaningful caring moments. Relationships develop and are to be celebrated.

Students' Freedom of Choice

Faculty members' efforts as teachers of nursing are governed by accreditation standards, curricular plans, and student-learning outcomes published in course syllabi. They create assignments to help students demonstrate their academic achievements in different courses. Faculty members' creative efforts are also seen as they meet students where they are. They shape course assignments with students as a way of encouraging, recognizing, and valuing student preferences and by encouraging the choice of topics significant to them in efforts to live the humanistic value, freedom of choice. An example is seen in a course on nursing research for evidence-based practice. The faculty member required approval of a research proposal topic as they wanted to avoid students' use of research papers that had been completed by a team in a hospital setting. One student shared that a team's study was soon to be published and that one author alone had written the review of literature section of the study. Since the student was interested in the study topic and needed to learn to write a research proposal independently, the nurse educator modified the research question in a discussion with the student. The student would benefit from all of the requirements specified in completing the proposal assignment. The student was pleased with her consultative decision, having been free to choose a preferred topic and demonstrating the value, freedom of choice.

Presence

Often at the beginning of courses and especially when getting down to the work required in the course, students share their discomfort about challenging courses and assignments. They fear failure. Faculty members display their understanding about how daunting course assignments can be, often repeating that they are accessible throughout the course and present to them, to answer questions and to clarify details of assignments. Faculty members show the caring attitude of being present.

A common practice at one school is to post blueprints on exams about 2 weeks before the test. Some also post several test questions on the learning management system for each module and hold, tape, and post asynchronous test sessions prior to midterm and final exams. In an online course, a faculty member scheduled sufficient time to answer test questions and also scheduled two sessions so that graduate students' work schedules were honored.

Compassion

Once in a course, a student scheduled for one session was admitted to a hospital for short-stay monitoring of her premature labor. The faculty member scheduled a single testing session for her. Displaying a compassionate attitude, the faculty member shares their view with graduate students that life happens and that they need to share stressful events with the faculty member. Few have taken advantage of the faculty member's flexibility. Rubrics that deconstruct assignments, such as papers, have also assisted students and nurse educators to clarify and visualize academic expectations.

Commitment and Availability

Faculty members' availability to students during a course is visible in various, often-used ways. Their commitment is seen when posting their availability in learning management systems by creating announcements that describe dates of conference attendance when away from the office. Their office hours are posted by office doors and frequently noted on syllabi; many describe that appointments can also be scheduled to be announced (TBA). Some make cell phone numbers available; a seasoned faculty member mentioned that, over many years of teaching, very few students used this access inappropriately. Accessible faculty members seem to "hover" over their courses, in a sense being consistently present to students and showing a caring attitude. Faculty members respond to text messages and emails in a timely fashion and apologize for delays, demonstrating once again their respect for students.

Mutual Trust

Students easily discern a nurse educator's enthusiasm for the content and processes of each course. This characteristic is frequently mentioned in course evaluations, whereby students describe faculty members' content knowledge and responsiveness to their concerns. The give-and-take between students and faculty members helps students to trust that faculty are invested in their success. Similarly, when students' performance is less than ideal, the faculty members' acceptance of students' critique of exam questions and paper comments provides an opportunity forum for mutual trust. In some schools, faculty members routinely analyze test item statistics and base grade adjustments made on items that do not perform well for test takers. Being reasonable, listening, and either applying or not applying credit for contentious questions and sharing decisions with students that may not please them, demonstrate that faculty members can be trusted. In such ways, faculty members display the caring attitudes of commitment to students' education and mutuality in the student–educator relationship.

Nurse Educators as Role Models: Part of the Hidden Curriculum
Finally, administrators and faculty members of schools of nursing as well as staff nurses and managers in clinical settings serve as role models for students (Karimi, Ashktorab, Mohammadi, & Abedi, 2014). As described (Chen, 2015), the parallel curriculum is collateral to the formal curriculum, and faculty members or clinical staff may not be aware of or intentional about it. Students pay attention to faculty members' and nurses' behavior, and other staff and professionals in both settings. They consider which behaviors to emulate and other actions to reject. The informal curriculum is a vehicle for teaching professionalism and consequently functions to socialize students into the professional role. Being more aware and intentional about the hidden curriculum provides an opportunity to emphasize caring principles.

CONCLUSION

This chapter intended to assist nurse educators to explore Human Caring values, attitudes, and behaviors in order to inform their learning/teaching practice and their relationships with their students, hence promoting their students' learning and development. Nurse educators' caring values, attitudes, and behaviors are paramount to accompany students in their learning journey of our discipline.

As Bevis (2000) strongly claims,

only a mentor / preceptor / teacher modeling a humanistically caring ethic and having dialogue with students that underscores constructed knowing and encourages them to be personally related to the ethical issues involved can facilitate and enhance students in their moral development for life and for nursing. (p. 184)

We believe that nurse educators, whose actions correspond to caring behaviors grounded in caring attitudes and values, have a caring moral ideal and a moral imperative guiding their teaching/learning praxis. Such a moral imperative transcends nurse educators' usual teaching role, guiding their leadership to humanize nursing education and raising their awareness to foster nursing's larger social mandate.

REFERENCES

Beck, C. T. (2001). Caring within nursing education: A metasynthesis. *Journal of Nursing Education, 40*(3), 101–109.

Bevis, E. O. (2000). Teaching and learning: The key to education and professionalism. In E. O. Bevis & J. Watson (Eds.), *Toward a caring curriculum: A new pedagogy for nursing* (2nd ed., pp. 153–188). London, UK: Jones & Bartlett.

Bevis, E. O., & Watson, J. (2000). *Toward a caring curriculum: A new pedagogy for nursing* (2nd ed.). London, UK: Jones & Bartlett.

Boeck, P. R. (2014, January–March). Presence: A concept analysis. *SAGE Open, 4*(1). doi:10.1177/2158244014527990

Boykin, A. (Ed.). (1994). *Living a caring-based program.* New York, NY: National League for Nursing Press.

Boykin, A., & Schoenhofer, S. O. (2001). *Nursing as caring: A model for transforming practice.* Sudbury, MA: Jones & Bartlett Publishers & National League for Nursing. (Original work published 1993)

Boykin, A., & Schoenhofer, S. O. (2013). Caring in nursing: Analysis of extant theory. In M. C. Smith, M. C. Turkel, & Z. Robinson Wolf (Eds.), *Caring in nursing classics: An essential resource* (pp. 33–42). New York, NY: Springer Publishing Company.

Cara, C. (2004, June). *Opening Keynote—Caring in 2004: Living it daily in our practice.* Keynote presented at the 26th Annual International Association for Human Caring Conference "Caring, for a Renewed Care", Montreal, QC, Canada.

Cara, C. (2017, June). *Rediscovering love, compassion, and caring to alleviate dehumanization.* Keynote speech at the 38th International Association for Human Caring Conference, Edmonton, AB, Canada.

Cara, C., Gauvin-Lepage, J., Lefebvre, H., Létourneau, D., Alderson, M., Larue, C., . . . Mathieu, C. (2016). Le Modèle humaniste des soins infirmiers—UdeM: Perspective novatrice et pragmatique. *Recherche en soins infirmiers, 125*, 20–31. doi:10.3917/rsi.125.0020

Cara, C., & Hills, M. (2018, May). *The added value of Caring Science: Its contributions to humanize nursing education.* Oral presentation at the Canadian Association of Schools in Nursing Conference, Montreal, QC, Canada.

Chan, E. A., Liu, J. Y. W, Fung, K. H. F., Tsang, P. L., & Yuen, J. (2018). Pre-departure preparation and co-curricular activities for students' intercultural exchange: A mixed-methods study. *Nurse Education Today, 63*, 43–49. doi:10.1016/j.nedt.2018.01.020

Chen, R. (2015). Commentary: Do as we say or do as we do? Examining the hidden curriculum in nursing education. *Canadian Journal of Nursing Research, 47*(3), 7–17. doi:10.1002/9781118883594.ch30

Devine, C. A., & Chin, E. D. (2018). Integrity in nursing students: A concept analysis. *Nurse Education Today, 60,* 133–138. doi:10.1016/j.nedt.2017.10.005

Duffy, J. R. (2018). *Quality caring in nursing and health systems* (3rd ed.). New York, NY: Springer Publishing Company.

Fawcett, J., & Chinn, P. (2019). *About.* Retrieved from https://nursology.net/about

Halldorsdottir, S. (1990). The essential structure of a caring and uncaring encounter with a teacher: The perspective of the nursing student. In M. Leininger & J. Watson (Eds.), *The caring imperative in nursing education* (pp. 95–108). New York, NY: National League for Nursing Press.

Hills, M., & Cara, C. (2019). Curriculum development processes and pedagogical practices for advancing Caring Science literacy. In W. Rosa, S. Horton-Deutsch, & J. Watson (Eds.), *A handbook for Caring Science: Expanding the paradigm* (pp. 197–210). New York, NY: Springer Publishing Company.

Hills, M., & Watson, J. (2011). *Creating a Caring Science curriculum: An emancipatory pedagogy for nursing.* New York, NY: Springer Publishing Company.

Karimi, Z., Ashktorab, T., Mohammadi, E., & Abedi, H. A. (2014). Using the hidden curriculum to teach professionalism in nursing students. *Iran Red Crescent Medical Journal, 16*(3), e155. doi:10.5812/ircmj.15532

Lazenby, M. (2017). *Caring matters most: The ethical significance of nursing.* New York, NY: Oxford University Press.

Lee, S., Palmieri, P., & Watson, J. (Eds.). (2017). *Global advances in Human Caring literacy.* New York, NY: Springer Publishing Company.

Mayeroff, M. (1971). *On caring.* New York, NY: Harper Perennial.

O'Reilly, L., Cara, C., & Delmas, P. (2016). Developing an educational intervention to strengthen the humanistic practices of hemodialysis nurses in Switzerland. *International Journal for Human Caring, 20*(1), 24–30. doi:10.20467/1091-5710-20.1.24

Ray, M. A. (2010). *Transcultural caring dynamics in nursing and health care.* Philadelphia, PA: F. A. Davis.

Roach, M. S. (2002). *Caring, the human mode of being: A blueprint for the health professions* (2nd ed.). Ottawa, ON, Canada: Cambridge Health Alliance Press.

Rosa, W., Horton-Deutsch, S., & Watson, J. (Eds). (2019). *A handbook for Caring Science: Expanding the paradigm.* New York, NY: Springer Publishing Company.

Smith, M. C., Turkel, M. C., & Wolf, Z. R. (Eds.). (2013). *Caring in nursing classics: An essential resource.* New York, NY: Springer Publishing Company.

Swanson, K. M. (2013). What is known about caring in nursing science: A literary meta-analysis. In M. C. Smith, M. C. Turkel & Z. R. Wolf (dir.) (Eds.), *Caring in nursing classics: An essential resource* (pp. 59–102). New York, NY: Springer Publishing Company.

Touhy, T., & Boykin, A. (2008). Caring as the central domain in nursing education. *International Journal of Human Caring, 12*(2), 8–15. doi:10.20467/1091-5710.12.2.8

Vachon, D. (2019). *How doctors care: The science of compassionate and balanced caring in medicine*. San Diego, CA: Cognella Academic Publishing.

van der Cingel, M. (2014). Compassion: The missing link in quality of care. *Nursing Education Today, 34*, 1253–1257. doi:10.1016/j.nedt.2014.04.003

Watson, J. (2008). *Nursing: The philosophy and science of caring* (revised ed.). Boulder: University Press of Colorado.

Watson, J. (2012). *Human Caring Science: A theory of nursing*. Sudbury, MA: Jones & Bartlett Learning.

Watson, J. (2018). *Unitary Caring Science: The philosophy and praxis of nursing*. Boulder: University Press of Colorado.

3

Emancipatory Contributions to Humanize Nursing Education: The Synergy of Critical Consciousness and Reflective Praxis

Without emancipation, education is an oppressive tool. It is an assembly-line industry producing nurse-workers who on average follow the status quo. They may make waves, but they stay within the rules while living lives that are circumscribed by the inflexibility of large medical empire-bureaucracies and bear the inevitable stamp of banality and mediocrity.
—Bevis, 2000a, pp. 162–163

LEARNING INTENTIONS

- Understand how nurse educators' critical consciousness contributes to humanize nursing education.
- Recognize the synergy between critical consciousness and reflective praxis.
- Explore how critical consciousness and reflective praxis create emancipatory education.

- Articulate the relationship between critical consciousness and reflective praxis to promote humanization in nursing education.
- Imagine how you as a nurse educator can develop your critical consciousness and reflective praxis to promote humanization of nursing education.

INTRODUCTION

Nursing education continues to embrace Freire's (1972) traditional "banking" approach to education, in which nurse educators view their students as vessels to be filled with information that the educators deem appropriate. For over 30 years, since the "curriculum revolution," we have recognized that nursing education must encourage critical consciousness, self-reflection, self-evaluation, and insight, which are attributes that are required to transform nursing; nevertheless, we often continue to reduce nursing education to oppressive behavioral and biomedical perspectives (Hills & Watson, 2011; National League for Nursing, 1988, 2003).

Freire's (2009) banking concept of education is reflected in the following beliefs and behaviors in nursing education:

- Nurse educators teach; students are taught.
- Nurse educators know everything; students know nothing.
- Nurse educators think; students are thought about.
- Nurse educators talk; students listen—meekly.
- Nurse educators discipline; students are disciplined.
- Nurse educators choose and enforce their choices; students comply.
- Nurse educators act; students have the illusion of acting through the action of teachers.
- Nurse educators choose program content; students learn it.
- Nurse educators confuse the authority of knowledge with their own professional authority, which they set in opposition to the freedom of their students.
- Nurse educators are the subject of the learning process; students are mere objects (adapted from Freire, 2009).

Now, over 30 years after the curriculum revolution, the question remains, *What will it take to overcome this pervasive nursing education perspective that has endured over 70 years of critique and scrutiny?* Can we unite around a desire to promote Caring Science and humanistic perspectives to finally overcome these dominant behaviorist perspectives?

In this chapter, we explore the path to a Relational Emancipatory Pedagogy for nursing education (Hills & Watson, 2011). We develop the argument for critical consciousness, reflective praxis, and emancipatory teaching strategies as the way forward to embrace this Relational Emancipatory Pedagogy, which helps to humanize nursing education. We include a Pragmatic Segment written by three graduate nursing students as an exemplar.

DEVELOPING NURSE EDUCATORS' CRITICAL CONSCIOUSNESS

In order to transcend these intransigent biomedical and behavioral perspectives of nursing education, we must begin with nurse educators' own development of self—becoming all they can be. Just as nurses have to develop themselves in order to recognize how important the "therapeutic use of self" is in nurse–patient relationships, nurse educators need to develop themselves in order to fully engage with students. This begins with nurse educators developing their own critical consciousness. Nurse educators' attempts to raise their consciousness require that they understand their world and its context and the influence that both their context and their sociopolitical history play in their day-to-day practice as educators. Critical consciousness, from a Freirean perspective, can be defined as

[t]he ability of individuals to take perspective on their immediate cultural, social, and political environment, to engage in critical dialogue with it, bringing to bear fundamental moral commitments including concerns for justice and equity, and to define their own place with respect to surrounding reality. (Mustakova-Possardt, 1998, p. 13)

For nurse educators, this means embracing caring as the moral imperative (of nursing) to act ethically and justly and teaching students to do the same (Hills & Watson, 2011).

As early as 1976, Smith operationalized Freire's concept of *conscientizacao* by describing three main existential tasks in the oppressor/oppressed relationship that must be resolved: naming the problem, reflecting on the problem, and acting on the problem. Mustakova-Possardt (1998) expands this description by examining the patterns of social interactions between social conditions and ordinary midlife individuals' experiences in the domains of work, family, social, and political life as well as moral and religious thinking. Mustakova-Possardt (1998) claims that through the exploration of these patterns of interactions of moral consciousness and adult development, we can understand how individuals may be led to the following:

- Question the set of social relations and the larger social environment in which they find themselves
- Feel compelled to make active efforts to transform their relationship with those social conditions in congruence with their understanding
- Seek an alternative vision of how things should be on grounds of explicit concerns with issues of justice and equity (p. 15)

She found that people who are critically conscious "problematize their social environment, bringing moral frames of reference to it. They often attempt to apply spiritual understanding to socio-political reality, and rely heavily on self-reflection in their efforts to bring inner and outer live[s] into harmony" (Mustakova-Possardt, 1998, p. 22).

For nurse educators, being critically conscious is essential in order for them to encourage and facilitate this development in their students. Nurse educators who are not critically conscious cannot engage with students in this emancipatory practice. If you are not critically conscious, you simply cannot give what you do not have, nor can you be who you are not. Students can usually tell those educators who are critically conscious and those who are not. Nurse educators living in a critically conscious manner in their daily lives will most likely encourage this way of being in their teaching of students.

Increasingly, graduating students are faced with entering complex and rapidly changing healthcare environments in which they are required to work autonomously. "[B]eing around others, especially those in roles of authority, with higher levels of critical consciousness may be the source of support for [critical consciousness] development" (Jemal, 2017, p. 614). Nurse educators must be able to think about their thinking; they need to be able to engage in this metacognition, which requires insight and the ability to participate in critically reflective thought processes. There is evidence that insight is required in order to participate in metacognition, "to think about one's own thoughts and emotions, links the present to the past, to provide a view for the future and to construct meaning of events" (Josephsen, 2014, p. 2).

So, how do we develop this critical consciousness in nursing education? Hills and Watson (2011) recommend that nurse educators, working from a critical conscious perspective, begin by aligning themselves with their students, not the content to be taught. As reflected in the "banking concept" of education, nurse educators often align themselves with the content and knowledge, viewing their students as receptacles to be filled with the information that the nurse educator decides is important to know. Working from a critical conscious perspective requires that nurse educators shift this thinking to understand the importance of first aligning with students and then together, in a caring relationship, the educator and the students engage with the content in a way that cocreates meaning and new knowledge. "This process of insight and integration with a deeper connection of meaning for 'personal knowing,' results in transformation of consciousness" (Hills & Watson, 2011, p. 53).

TIME OUT FOR REFLECTION

The authors invite you to write your reflection in a journal in order to link the preceding theoretical segment with your personal journey as a nurse educator.

Think about a time when you experienced being "critically conscious," and then ask yourself the following questions:

- Who was involved?
- What were the characteristics illustrating your critical consciousness?
- Describe the context of the situation that heightened your awareness?
- What was going on in the environment that triggered your attention?
- Describe your experience in your journal and share this experience with your colleagues.

Nurses, and specifically nurse educators, who embrace Human Caring as the theoretical, philosophical, and ethical foundation of nursing must also embrace caring as the moral imperative to act ethically and justly. In other words, for these nurse educators, caring is their moral compass when making decisions for appropriate, just, and ethical actions.

In addition, nurse educators who are critically conscious can recognize the hegemony both in daily clinical nursing practice and in nursing education practice. "Hegemony refers to the maintenance of domination not by the sheer exercise of force but primarily through consensual social practices, social forms, and social structures produced in specific sites such as the church, the state, the school, the media, the political system, and the family" (McLaren,

2009, p. 67). When nurse educators are aware of hegemony, they are able to articulate counterhegemony strategies to disrupt hegemonic power, and they can discuss these strategies with their students. This understanding by nurse educators encourages students to further develop their critical consciousness, question taken-for-granted assumptions, initiate change, and transform undemocratic, authoritarian behaviors and attitudes into caring attitudes and behaviors.

Because nursing is a practice-based discipline, nurse educators also need to be aware of hegemony in nursing practice so they can assist students to identify it in their clinical experiences and question them. An antiquated example from early nursing practice was the action of the nurse when a physician entered the nursing station. The nurse would stand and give the physician her chair. No one told the nurse to do so, but it was expected. It becomes common practice and the status quo.

An example of hegemony in nursing education is apparent in the way we choose to structure the classroom. When we line up the desks or use a classroom with fixed chairs, we are engaged in a "power-over," educator-controlled situation, where we are saying (without saying a word) that the teacher is in control. This sends the message that the teacher has the knowledge and that students are expected to listen and absorb what the educator says. The same can be said of multiple-choice exams. The nurse educator decides what information is to be learned and the student is expected to regurgitate the information that the educator has decided is to be learned. These hegemonic practices usually go unnoticed by the nurse educator or the students. They are accepted as what commonly happens in an education setting. From a Human Caring perspective, there is no room for dominant–passive power relationships. Power relations need to be discussed and negotiated. It may not be possible to eradicate all power-over situations in nursing education, but it is possible to discuss them with students, which raises their consciousness and moves them to a state of greater awareness. "Understanding how hegemony functions in society provides [nurse educators] with the basis of understanding not only how the seeds of domination are produced, but also how they can be challenged and overcome through resistance, critique and social action" (Darder, Baltodano, & Torres, 2009, p. 12).

It is important to note that critical consciousness is not only about individual self-awareness, insight, or empowerment. Critical consciousness has a sociopolitical aspect to it (see also Chapter 8, Nurse Educators' Political Caring Literacy and Power to Promote Caring Relationships in Nursing Education). As Shor and Freire (1987) explain, even when you feel yourself most free, if this feeling is not a social feeling, if you are not able to use your recent freedom to help others to be free by transforming the totality of society, then you are exercising an individualistic attitude towards empowerment and freedom. (p. 109)

It takes courage to address inequities, speak to hegemony, create counterhegemony, and speak truth to power. It is easier to adapt—to be quiet, to mind your own business, or claim to be neutral. We see this with nurse educators who recognize dehumanizing practices (see Chapter 1, Grounded in a Human Science Paradigm) but remain silent. To humanize nursing education, nurse educators must speak out when they observe dehumanizing practices. "Emancipatory education encourages learners [and teachers] to ask the unaskable, confront injustices and oppression, and be active agencies in their lives and work" (Hills & Watson, 2011, p. 55).

TIME OUT FOR REFLECTION

The authors invite you to write your reflection in a journal in order to link the preceding theoretical segment with your personal teaching/learning experiences.

Think about a time when you recognized a dehumanizing hegemonic practice but did not speak up, and then ask yourself the following questions:

- Who was involved?
- What were the characteristics of the situation that made it hegemonic?
- What stopped you from speaking up?
- How did you feel (positive and negative feelings) in this situation?

Now think of a time when you recognized a dehumanizing hegemonic situation and you did speak up, and then ask yourself these questions:

- Who was involved?
- What were the characteristics that made the situation hegemonic?
- How did you feel (positive and negative feelings) when you spoke up?
- How can Human Caring be linked with the fact that you spoke up about this dehumanizing hegemonic situation?
- How was this situation different than the one described earlier?

REFLECTIVE PRAXIS

Reflection is a key process in learning, and there are several ways to engage students in this process. Nurse educators frequently provide opportunities for students to reflect on their experiences such as in postconference debriefing sessions or at critical points in classroom-learning situations. Reflection, reflectivity, and the concept of the reflective practitioner have gained prominence in nursing education since Schön's (1983) introduction of the concept in his doctoral dissertation as a student of Dewey. Nursing education has fully embraced this concept of reflection and continues to praise its significance in nursing to this day (Nelson, 2012; Josephsen, 2014). Moreover, as Horton-Deutsch and Cara (2017) explained, reflective practice is in coherence with Human Caring in nursing education, as it invites students to reflect on their future practice and how to improve the quality of care they provide to their patients.

We highlight different ways that reflection is discussed in nursing education (see also Chapter 7, Habitus: An Ontological Space Fostering Humanistic Nursing Education) and distinguish among various aspects of reflective praxis in nursing education.

Reflection-on-Action and Experiences

Nurse educators need to deliberately engage in reflection and reflective processes. Boud, Keogh, and Walker (1985) state that "reflection in the context of learning is a generic term for those intellectual and affective activities in which individuals engage to explore their experiences in order to lead to new understandings and appreciations" (p. 19). This type of reflection is almost always considered internal and isolated individual experiences. Drawing from Boud et al. (1985) as well as Hills and Watson (2011), we conclude that nurse educators are the only ones who can reflect on their own intentions and experiences of teaching.

Based on Dewey's five aspects of reflection, Boud et al. (1985) developed a three-stage model explicating three essential aspects of this reflective process. When considered in nurse educators' teaching practice, these include:

1. Returning to the experience: Nurse educators are prompted to recall salient features; recollecting the experience can create insight.
2. Attending to feelings: Nurse educators are encouraged to identify positive and negative feelings. Nurse educators are invited to use

their positive feelings to overcome what might be a challenging teaching situation.

3. Reevaluating the experience: Experience is reexamined in relation to nurse educators' intent. New knowledge is integrated into nurse educators' conceptual framework.

This final phase involves four processes: association, integration, validation, and appropriation. Through these processes, nurse educators realize disparities between older and newer ways of thinking, integrate new ways of knowing, synthesize new information, test their new ideas, and develop personal meaning of the new knowledge.

This type of reflection is taught and used extensively in nursing education programs to enhance students' reflective capacities and develop insight. Here, we are recommending that nurse educators use these processes to develop their own capacities. This type of reflection can lead to change through increased understanding, awareness, and insight. However, another type of reflection, reflection-in-action, is key for nurse educators and is related to critical consciousness. Reflection-in-action always leads to transformational change (Hills & Watson, 2011).

Reflection-in-Action: Emancipatory Praxis

Schön (1983) advances reflection in nursing education with his introduction of the concept of the "reflective practitioner." As a practice-based discipline, nursing quickly embraced this concept in nursing education (Hills & Watson, 2011; Kinsella, 2010). We are recommending that it is also a useful and necessary capability for nurse educators. Schön claims that this ability is an intuitive, creative, artistic process and much more than the cognitive/affective process described earlier by Boud. As Schön (1983) explains,

> when we go about the spontaneous, intuitive performance of actions of life, we show ourselves to be knowledgeable in a special way . . . our knowing is ordinarily tacit, implicit in our pattern of action and in our feel for the stuff with which we are dealing. It seems right to say our knowledge is in our action. (p. 49)

This type of reflection, reflection-in-action, is similar to Benner and Wrubel's (1989) foundational research that illuminated "tacit knowledge" in nursing practice. This type of reflection is as critical in nursing education as it is in practice because no matter how well prepared we are, teaching/ facilitating dialogue often demands that we *think on our feet*. We must be able to think about what we are doing, saying, or thinking while we are doing it! This implies that we must have critical consciousness, as described earlier, in order to engage in this type of reflection.

Kemmis (1985) advances this concept of reflection-in-action and further links it to critical consciousness by adding political, emancipatory, and social aspects to this conceptualization of reflection. As he explains, "reflection is a political act which hastens or defers the realization of a more rational, just and fulfilling society" (p. 140). For nurse educators who understand the synergy of critical consciousness and reflective praxis, they need to commit to continuing to develop these attitudes and skills in the political and social contexts in which they find themselves (See also Chapter 8, Nurse Educators' Political Caring Literacy and Power to Promote Caring Relationships in Nursing Education).

This conceptualization of reflection recognizes the inextricable link between theory and action, which is praxis. It views knowledge as a dialectic (Hills & Watson, 2011). As Darder et al. (2009) explain, "all human activity is understood as emerging from ongoing interactions of reflection, dialogue and action—namely praxis—and as praxis, all human activity requires theory to illuminate it and provide a better understanding of the world as we find it and as it might be" (p. 13). For nurse educators, this means understanding the theory that they use in teaching and reflecting on their actual way of teaching to understand its congruence with the theory they espouse. In other terms, it means that their words are congruent with their actions. If nurse educators claim Caring teaching practices but do not act on them, they have no claim to being a Caring Science educator.

What is so compelling about this conception of praxis is the inherent expectation to initiate change. For nurse educators, this means recognizing humanizing practices and changing their teaching to embrace these practices. A change in actions and theory is an expected outcome. It suggests a continuing unfolding of creation, creativity, and learning. Kemmis (1985) explains it this way:

> [Reflection] looks inward at our thoughts and thought processes and outward at the situation in which we find ourselves; when we consider the interaction of internal and external, our reflection orients us for further thought and action. Thus, reflection is meta thinking—thinking about thinking in which we consider the relationship between our thoughts and actions in a particular context. (p. 40)

Currently, there is a tendency in nursing programs to focus almost exclusively on competency-based outcomes or standards-of-practice models to prepare students for practice. Unfortunately, these models often tend to limit teaching to behaviors that can be measured while ignoring critical aspects of emancipation such as self-awareness, insight, compassion, and caring, as well as other attributes of reflective and caring praxis.

> It can be argued that the focus on solely competency based curricular theory, that is enmeshed in the rational and behavioristic approaches to knowledge development and integration, has led to a curricular focus in nursing education that ignores the essential aspects of self-awareness and reflexivity in knowledge formation. (Josephsen, 2014, p. 2)

We would add that this is true for nurse educators as well as students. This focus on competencies or standards of practice in isolation leads nurse educators to often ignore some of the most foundational aspects of nursing such as critical consciousness, metacognition, comforting, and alleviating suffering. Most competencies focus on behaviors that are quantifiable and can be measured. However, as Hills and Watson (2011) as well as Hills and Cara (2019) explain, many critical aspects of nursing cannot be measured. Furthermore, Bevis (2000b) specifically identifies "intuition, insight, caring, compassion, reflection, creativity, or flexibility" (p. 266) as being significant attributes for nurses that cannot be measured. She raises the question "how can one be confident in his or her competence to evaluate the student's ability to see patterns, find meaning and significance, see balance and wholeness, identify with the ethical and cultural traditions of the discipline, and so on?" (p. 266).

Thus, as nurse educators, we are left with the challenge to prepare our students not only with nursing skills and knowledge but also with the internal skills of self-evaluation, reflexivity, self-awareness, insight, critical thinking, and decision-making processes, as well as to instill the values of the discipline, which include caring, social justice, and equity (Hills & Cara, 2019; Hills & Watson, 2011; Josephsen, 2014). "As nursing evolves its disciplinary foundation, it is time to stand in this base and claim those invisible aspects of nursing as core to our practice and therefore to nursing education" (Hills, 2017, cited in Hills & Cara, 2019, p. 199). Furthermore, if we do not evaluate students on these critical aspects of Human Caring in nursing, they will go unnoticed and remain invisible.

To meet this challenge, nurse educators need to provide opportunities for students to have actual practice experiences in which they can learn to reflect-in-action. Doing so makes these critical aspects *visible* to discuss, to capture in reflective journals, and to "matter" as expected nursing actions.

TIME OUT FOR REFLECTION

The authors invite you to write your reflection in a journal in order to link the preceding theoretical segment with your personal teaching/learning experiences.

They invite you to consider the following questions:

- What strategies do you/can you do to enhance your critical consciousness?
- How can you, as a nurse educator, enhance your reflection-in-action capacities?
- What caring strategies can you use in the classroom to humanize students' learning experiences?
- What caring strategies can you use to humanize clinical teaching?
- Do you use humanistic teaching strategies? If so, what are they?

Share your strategies in your next small group discussion.

You might want to begin to develop a repository of different teaching strategies that you can use to humanize students' experiences.

PRAGMATIC SEGMENT
CREATING A CRITICAL RELATIONAL CARING FRAMEWORK: STUDENTS' LIVED EXPERIENCE IN A RELATIONAL EMANCIPATORY PEDAGOGY

Jessica Eitel, MN, BSN, RNC-NIC, Benita Lee, MN, BScN, RN, CPN(C), and Ruhina Rana, MN, BSN, BA, RN

Background

As part of a graduate nursing course grounded in Relational Emancipatory Pedagogy, future nurse educators were asked to work in groups to develop a conceptual pedagogical framework. This endeavor, created by our nurse educator, challenged students to develop critical consciousness while working synergistically to actualize reflective praxis. This Pragmatic Segment describes the transformation that occurs when learners are truly engaged in the process of cocreated learning.

Our framework was developed through Hills and Watson's (2011) Caring Science lens, with all contributors actively engaged and embracing

Relational Emancipatory Pedagogy. Initial discussions among members revealed a shared affinity for Freire's work (1972), thus enabling the group to articulate a collective critical consciousness as the foundation for the endeavor. Subsequently, we were able to readily identify a group philosophy and define related concepts, which would become the elements of our framework.

This framework is representative of a genuinely collaborative process. We started with three distinct philosophies and, in respectfully sharing our individual pedagogies, were able to articulate strengths and acknowledge limitations to develop a collective framework. As we sought to develop a framework that supports transformative learning, we were cognizant of modeling the principles of Caring Science in our own interactions. Indeed, our collaborative processes were largely shaped by the essential components we identified as creating collaborative caring relationships, engaging in critical caring dialogue, and reflecting-in-action (Kemmis, 1985). Our group's process demonstrated that reflection-in-action, and specifically Caring Science *in* praxis, correlated directly with the synergistic manifestation of a pedagogical framework that is aligned with a Caring Science Curriculum.

Creating a Group Framework

At the onset of this assignment, our group members committed to approach this project respectfully, consciously, and critically to develop a pedagogical framework that was reflective of a cohesive philosophical perspective. As part of a distance education program, we found it valuable to schedule weekly video chats throughout the course of our work to facilitate a more personal exchange in addition to email communication and shared documents. We believe that this humanizing aspect strongly supported our cohesiveness as a group, enabling us to connect on a personal and more meaningful level.

We grounded our process in the very elements of Caring Science we hoped to build upon in our own pedagogical framework: building caring relationships and engaging in critical reflective dialogue (Hills & Watson, 2011). We were then able to articulate a group philosophical perspective, with a shared view on curriculum, teaching, and learning. As a result, a cohesive pedagogical framework evolved quite naturally, reflecting our ethics of caring, our critical consciousness, and our support for transformative learning. We called this framework Critical Relational Caring (see Figure 3.1).

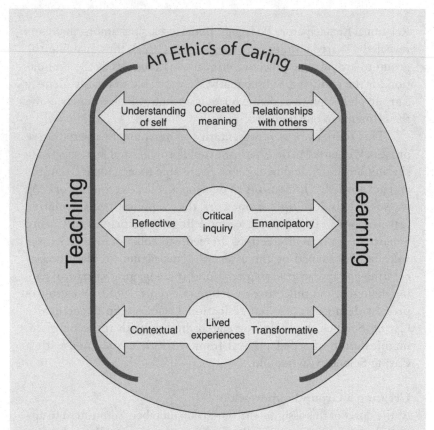

Figure 3.1 Critical Relational Caring (CRC) framework diagram.
Source: Adapted from Hills, M., & Watson, J. (2011). *Creating a caring curriculum: An emancipatory pedagogy for nursing.* New York, NY: Springer Publishing Company.

Critical Relational Caring Framework

In our Critical Relational Caring (CRC) framework, as within Hills and Watson's (2011) Caring Science Curriculum, the relationship between learning and teaching is to create meaningful experiences that enable learners to make connections between nursing knowledge and theory as well as between social contexts and professional practice.

The first content theme within our framework is *cocreated meaning* (see Figure 3.1). Within our multipedagogical approach, cocreated meaning is balanced between the subthemes of the *nurse educator's and students' understanding of self* and their *relationship with others*. It is imperative to create a learning environment where students and nurse educators can be coinvested to develop and share knowledge that engages their moral beliefs of caring (Hills & Watson, 2011).

Using Critical Social Theory (Freire, 1972; Josephsen, 2014) and Emancipatory Relational Pedagogy (Hills & Watson, 2011), the second theme, *critical inquiry*, is fundamental to develop innovative teaching and learning approaches that are designed to encourage and involve students to become responsible and engaged learners (Brown, Kirkpatrick, Greer, Matthias, & Swanson, 2009). Using Hills and Watson's (2011) Caring Science Curriculum as the philosophical and pedagogical underpinning for our framework, we utilize the subthemes of *reflective* and *emancipatory* practices. Using this perspective, nurse educators can create trusting relationships and a culture where critical dialogue is encouraged (Hills & Watson, 2011). We believe that this interactive process for learning through critical inquiry creates meaningful personal growth and frames the development of knowledge within context.

The final content theme of our CRC framework is based on the *lived experiences* within the teacher–student–environment intersection that provides *transformative* and *contextual* learning. As students are engaged in their personal learning, nurse educators share the power and responsibility to promote lived experiences that will enable students to connect nursing knowledge with real-life contexts. Our pedagogical framework promotes an inclusive, open, flexible, and holistic environment that encourages students to critically reflect on their experiences and create meaningful perceptions in the ethics of caring (Watson, 1999). As the ethics of caring encircles the framework (see Figure 3.1) around the nursing content, contexts, and moral imperatives, the nursing curriculum can be developed to transform learners to be safe and caring professionals (Hills & Watson, 2011). We believe that our CRC framework is an emancipatory approach to developing curriculum that enables teachers and learners alike to bring the ethics of caring and context of lived experience to professional nursing practice.

Critical Relational Caring and Caring Science
The four elements of the Relational Emancipatory Pedagogy (Hills & Watson, 2011) are visually represented in the interlocking circles of our framework. Caring Science frames the essential components of creating "collaborative caring relationships," engaging in "critical caring dialogue," and "reflecting-in-action" within an overarching

emancipatory relational concept of "creating a culture of caring" (Hills & Watson, 2011, p. 69). Similarly, our framework embraces caring as an ethic that transcends nursing education and nursing practice through the understanding that people are interconnected and holistic beings who derive meaning through critical inquiry, relationships, and lived experiences. In our framework, the ethics of caring encapsulate the themes and the corresponding subthemes that constitute our framework (see Figure 3.1).

Our framework for teaching and learning in nursing education aligns with many of the tenets of Caring Science. Hills and Watson (2011) hold creating caring relationships as critical to Relational Emancipatory Pedagogy. Our framework also maintains that relationships with others contribute to one's understanding of self and are thus integral to the development of cocreated meaning. The relationship between the nurse educator and students is built on trust, self-reflection, and personal meaning within academia and social contexts (Hills & Watson, 2011). In Caring Science, critical dialogue creates "opportunities for critical thinking and critical reflection that result in the creation of new understandings (knowledge)" (Hills & Watson, 2011, p. 88). In our framework, critical inquiry embraces a reflective emancipatory process that facilitates decentralized and empowered engagement in learning by testing ideas, challenging assumptions, and thoughtfully navigating problems. Hills and Watson (2011) present reflection-in-action as the experiential component of transformational learning and teaching. In a related perspective, our framework views lived experiences as a primary theme; these experiences are informed by context and have the potential to generate transformative learning and humanize nursing education.

Evaluation

The CRC framework supports the use of evaluations as "landmarks" to give both students and nurse educators an indication of where they stand in relation to where they plan to go within a course (Hills & Watson, 2011). In this sense, it is important to consider assessment as a means but not an end in transformational learning (Hills & Watson, 2011). As the teaching and learning pillars focus on the subthemes of "cocreated meaning," "critical inquiry," and "lived experiences," we believe that evaluation methods should focus on the process and progress toward these ends in view, but not necessarily the ends in and of themselves. Also, it is imperative that evaluation criteria focus on elements that are nursing-focused (carative) versus medically focused (curative) (Hills & Watson, 2011).

Conclusion
Our CRC framework utilizes various teaching, learning, and evaluation strategies that are in keeping with our philosophical position based on Hills and Watson's (2011) Relational Emancipatory Pedagogy grounded in Caring Science. Our conceptual pedagogical framework is dynamic and evolving. It will require reflection and reevaluation to ensure the curriculum based on it remains true to its philosophical and theoretical underpinnings and meets the needs of both teachers and learners.

CONCLUSION

In this chapter, we explored the contributions of emancipation to humanize nursing education. As discussed, critical consciousness and reflective praxis create an evolving and transforming nursing education in a more humane environment so that students' learning can be meaningful. In particular, we described the synergy of critical consciousness and reflective praxis as being significant aspects of nurse educators' perspectives to humanize nursing education.

REFERENCES

Benner, P., & Wrubel, J. (1989). *The primacy of caring.* Menlo Park, CA: Addison-Wesley.

Bevis, E. (2000a). Teaching and learning: The Key to education and professionalism. In E. Bevis & J. Watson (Eds.), *Towards a caring curriculum: Towards a new pedagogy for nursing* (pp. 153–188). New York, NY: National League for Nursing.

Bevis, E. (2000b). Accessing learning: Determining worth or developing excellence—From a behaviorist toward an interpretive-criticism model. In E. Bevis & J. Watson (Eds.), *Towards a caring curriculum: Towards a new pedagogy for nursing* (pp. 261–303). New York, NY: National League for Nursing.

Boud, D., Keogh, R., & Walker, D. (Eds.). (1985). *Reflection: Turning experience into learning.* London, UK: Kogan Page.

Brown, S., Kirkpatrick, M., Greer, A., Matthias, A., & Swanson, M. (2009). The use of innovative pedagogies in nursing education: An international perspective. *Nurse Education Perspectives, 30*(3), 153–158.

Darder, A., Baltodano, M., & Torres, R. (2009). Critical pedagogy: An introduction. In A. Darder, M. Baltodano, & R. Torres (Eds.), *The critical pedagogy reader* (pp. 1–20). New York, NY: Routledge.

Freire, P. (1972). *Pedagogy of the oppressed*. London, UK: Penguin Books.

Freire, P. (2009). From pedagogy of the oppressed. In A. Darder, M. Baltodano, & R. Torres (Eds.), *The critical pedagogy reader* (pp. 52–60). New York, NY: Routledge.

Hills, M., & Cara, C. (2019). Curriculum development processes and pedagogical practices for advancing Caring Science literacy. In W. Rosa, S. Horton-Deutsch, & J. Watson (Eds.), *A handbook for Caring Science: Expanding the paradigm* (pp. 197–210). New York, NY: Springer Publishing Company.

Hills, M., & Watson, J. (2011). *Creating a caring curriculum: An emancipatory pedagogy for nursing*. New York, NY: Springer Publishing Company.

Horton-Deutsch, S., & Cara, C. (2017). Learning through reflection and reflection on learning: Pedagogies in action. In S. Horton-Deutsch & G. D. Sherwood (Eds.), *Reflective practice: Transforming education and improving outcomes* (2nd ed., pp. 137–166). Indianapolis, IN: Sigma Theta Tau International.

Jemal, A. (2017). Critical consciousness: A critique and critical analysis of the literature. *Urban Review, 49*(4), 602–626. doi:10.1007/s11256-017-0411-3

Josephsen, J. (2014). Critically reflexive theory: A proposal for nursing education. *Advances in Nursing, 2014*, 594360, 7 p. doi:10.1155/2014/594360

Kemmis, S. (1985). Action research and the politics of reflection. In D. Boud, R. Keogh, & D. Walker (Eds.), *Reflection: Turning experience into learning* (pp. 139–164). London, UK: Kogan Page.

Kinsella, E. A. (2010). Professional knowledge and the epistemology of reflective practice. *Nursing Philosophy, 11*(1), 3–14. doi:10.1111/j.1466-769X.2009.00428.x

McLaren, P. (2009). Critical pedagogy: A look at the major concepts. In A. Darder, M. Baltodano, & R. Torres (Eds.), *The critical pedagogy reader* (2nd ed., pp. 52–60). New York, NY: Routledge.

Mustakova-Possardt, E. (1998). Critical consciousness: An alternative pathway for positive personal and social development. *Journal of Adult Development, 5*(1), 13–30. doi:10.1023/A:1023064913072

National League for Nursing. (1988). *Curriculum revolution: A mandate for change*. New York, NY: National League for Nursing.

National League for Nursing. (2003). *Position statement. Innovation in nursing education: A call to reform*. Retrieved from http://www.nln.org/docs/default-source/about/archived-position-statements/innovation-in-nursing-education-a-call-to-reform-pdf.pdf

Nelson, S. (2012). The lost path to emancipatory practice: Towards a history of reflective practice in nursing. *Nursing Philosophy, 13*(3), 202–213. doi:10.1111/j.1466-769X.2011.00535.x

Schön, D. (1983). *The reflective practitioner: How professionals think in action*. New York, NY: Basic Books.

Shor, I., & Freire, P. (1987). *A pedagogy for liberation: Dialogues on transforming education*. Westport, CT: Bergin & Garvey.

Smith, W. A. (1976). *The meaning of conscientizacao: The goal of Paolo Freire's pedagogy*. Amherst: Center for International Education, University of Massachusetts.

Watson, J. (1999). *Postmodern nursing and beyond*. Edinburgh, UK: Churchill Livingstone.

4

Humanizing Nursing Education by Teaching From the Heart

A good educator is not content driven, but driven by love, by passion, intellect, moral ideas, by your desire to inspire students to reach the highest level of their potential, even when they cannot see or believe in themselves.
—Watson, 2018a, p. 189

LEARNING INTENTIONS

- Sensitize nurse educators about the importance of teaching from the heart to humanize nursing education and facilitate students' learning.
- Reflect on teaching from the heart as an act of caring and an act of love.
- Appreciate the added value of teaching from the heart, for both students and nurse educators.
- Understand, from the nurse educator's perspective, what it is like to be teaching from the heart.

INTRODUCTION

In this chapter, after looking at the prevalent nurse educator's role, we reflect on the importance, for nurse educators, to be *teaching from the heart* and how it can contribute to humanize nursing education as well as facilitate students' learning. The added value of teaching from the heart, for students and nurse educators alike, is also discussed. In addition, a Pragmatic Segment illustrates these ideas more concretely.

THE NURSE EDUCATOR'S TEACHING ROLE

We briefly discuss the nurse educator's teaching role. Even though Hunt (2018) describes other roles for the nurse educator, such as "service" and "scholarship," we concentrate, for the purpose of this book, on the "teaching" role. According to Benner, Sutphen, Leonard, and Day (2010), the clinical instructor and the academical nurse educator may have very different roles. Yet, in agreement with Hunt (2018), we consider that both are involved in "teaching" students to become nurses, as an utmost responsibility. Therefore, we believe that teaching from the heart can be valuable to both academic and clinical nurse educators.

The teaching role of nurse educators implies that they develop or revise course syllabi, determine important reading materials, develop course out-lines and assignments, use different teaching strategies to teach students, be a role model, guide students in their learning process, evaluate students' learning, and so forth. Moreover, this teaching role will develop over time and depends on each educator's experiences as well as their knowledge. In other words, nurse educators develop their own unique style, which is influenced not only by their own personal beliefs, pedagogies, and styles but also from the beliefs, pedagogies, and philosophy of their academic institution (Hunt, 2018). Therefore, if a nursing school has selected to implement a Caring Curriculum, as proposed, for example, by Hills and Watson (2011), it may assist nurse educators to be informed by a Human Caring perspective in their teaching role.

Hence, we can ask the following questions: How will nurse educators be informed by a Human Caring perspective? What will then be different in their teaching role? Needless to say, we are convinced that a Human Caring perspective can be a significant foundation to learn to "teach from the heart," along with contributing to humanize nursing education.

EXPANDING THE TEACHING ROLE: TEACHING FROM THE HEART AS AN ACT OF CARING

We believe that the nurse educator's "teaching role" should not be limited to the preceding tasks, even though they are necessary to perform as an educator. Rather, the nurse educator's teaching role should include creating a safe space for students to learn, supporting and accompanying students throughout their learning process, as well as inviting questions and dialogue about the content and the proposed assignment. In other words, we are convinced that the nurse educator's teaching role should be an "act of caring."

If caring is the core of our discipline, it should then be central to the entire profession, in this case, the education realm. Consequently, Human Caring, as an ontology (i.e., meaning the nature of being and our existence), can inform the nurse educator's teaching role, inviting teaching to become a "relational human process." In other words, Human Caring can provide an ontological perspective for nurse educators to focus on students' learning as well as students–educators caring relationships. Thereby, the following questions become relevant: What is the nature of being and becoming a caring teacher? What is the nature of teaching from a Human Caring perspective? As Hills and Watson (2011) eloquently mention, "as we nursing educators begin to embrace Caring Science as a philosophical and theoretical foundation upon which to teach nursing, we must embrace a pedagogy that is congruent with this orientation" (p. 55). Teaching from the heart is such an orientation. But what exactly is teaching from the heart?

Teaching From the Heart: Its Meaning

We strongly believe that teaching from the heart is based on the nurse educator's ethical responsibility, moral imperative, as well as commitment to facilitate students' acquisition of knowledge related to being and becoming caring competent nurses. First, it is an ethical responsibility as the nurse educator's beliefs of doing what is morally right. Thus, it goes beyond simply giving students the course's content. Moreover, as nurse educators, it is our moral imperative (aiming to be the best nurse educator that is possible) that allows us to guide and support our students to understand what it means to be a caring nurse. As Watson (2018b) explains, a moral imperative is necessary to uphold Human Caring as well as human integrity, wholeness, and dignity. Lastly, it originates from the nurse educator's commitment to walk alongside students to facilitate their integration of knowledge and skills. Boykin and Schoenhofer (2013) have defined "commitment" as the nurse's embodiment of his or her function and ethic. Consequently, for these reasons, teaching from the heart becomes vital to humanize nursing education.

Additionally, teaching from the heart implies that teachers accompany students in their journey toward learning, success, and emancipation. As Hills and Watson (2011) explain, learning takes place within the student–teacher caring relationship, where they are cocreating knowledge. In order to do so, Hills and Watson acknowledge that an emancipatory pedagogy, instead of a traditional pedagogy, will promote the students' transformation of consciousness (see also Chapter 3, Emancipatory Contributions to Humanize Nursing Education) in order for learning and deeper insights to arise. "Transformation of consciousness includes an evolution of consciousness, in that both student and teacher experience a higher dimension of integration from before, including a higher consciousness and repatterning of old into something new" (Hills & Watson, 2011, p. 54).

Furthermore, teaching from the heart is showing oneself as a human being, allowing oneself, as a nurse educator, to reveal yourself to students and to the domain you are teaching. In order to do that, you need to know yourself. As Palmer (1997) explains,

> *good teaching cannot be reduced to technique; good teaching comes from the identity and integrity of the teacher.* . . . My ability to connect with my students, and to connect them with the subject, depends less on the methods I use than on the degree to which I know and trust my selfhood—and am willing to make it available and vulnerable in the service of learning. (p. 2)

Nevertheless, Vitali (2017, 2019) argues that the phenomenon teaching from the heart has not been present in the nursing literature. She reports finding this surprising since the nursing discipline has been studying empathy and caring for several years. From an empirical standpoint, Vitali's (2017, 2019) qualitative phenomenological and narrative inquiry demonstrated that 10 nursing teachers from the United States and Canada described their experience of "teaching from the heart." From her participants' stories, she has identified the following six themes (these themes are exemplified in the Pragmatic Segment):

- Experiencing a hard job
- Knowing and living caring
- Embracing vulnerability
- Learning and growing together
- Being in right relationship
- Experiencing spiritual transformation (Vitali, 2019, p. 237).

Said differently, Vitali's (2017, 2019) research results have shown that teaching from the heart means that teachers need to consider students as whole human beings filled with wisdom, entering in the student–teacher relationship, as well as sharing one's vulnerability. Finally, inspired by Watson's work, Vitali (2017) suggests that teaching from the heart corresponds to transpersonal caring/healing experiences for teachers, guided by Human Caring.

In other words, Human Caring can inform the nurse educator's teaching role to humanize nursing education. Not only are we convinced that the nurse educator's teaching role should be an "act of caring," but we are persuaded that it should be an "act of love." But one could ask: What does *love* have to do with nursing education or the nurse educator's role?

EXPANDING THE TEACHING ROLE: TEACHING FROM THE HEART AS AN ACT OF LOVE

The Meaning of Love in the Nursing Discipline

The concept of "love" is hardly seen in the nursing literature. Fitzgerald (1998), Goldin (2016), and Stickley and Freshwater (2002) have suggested different rationales to explain why "love" is rarely found in our nursing literature. For instance, according to these authors, love has several meanings without reaching any consensus (e.g., affection, maternal love, romantic love, or altruistic or unselfish love); love has been associated with "romance," which is being perceived as professionally unacceptable; or simply, the word *love* is "taboo" in nursing, and therefore it should not be used.

Empirically, Swanson's (2013) results of her meta-analysis on "caring in nursing" indicate that "love" was not reported directly; however, the term "loving" did appear, but not frequently. A few authors (Fitzgerald, 1998; Goldin, 2016, 2017, 2019; Stickley & Freshwater, 2002; Thorkildsen, Eriksson, & Raholm, 2013, 2015) have explored or reflected upon the different meanings of "love": "eros," which corresponds to romantic love; "agape," which means unconditional love; or "Caritas," which relates to altruistic love or loving-kindness. These authors conclude that "love" in nursing is usually linked to "agape" or "Caritas" (Goldin, 2017, 2019; Stickley & Freshwater, 2002; Thorkildsen et al., 2013, 2015).

For example, using Eriksson's Caring Science theory in their interpretative research synthesis to explore love when experiencing suffering, Thorkildsen et al. (2013) conclude that "love can be understood as agape . . . . expressed through the ethical responsibility inviting the suffering human in to a communion where suffering can be shared" (p. 458). More recently, Goldin (2017, 2019), in her hermeneutical study on love with ICU nurses, also discusses love as "agape" and concludes that love strengthens Caring

Science, taking it to a deeper level. For Goldin (2019), love corresponds to a dynamic human energy, which touches both patients' and nurses' souls and spirit. On the other hand, Watson (2017) connects love with "Caritas." She defines love as "the highest level of consciousness" (p. 226), "a form of Unitive energy processed by the heart which brings all of life together" (p. 237), and "as the ethical values foundation of health care" (p. 228).

Despite the fact that different authors link "love" with the term "agape" or the term "Caritas," if love is vital to our humanity, it might then be relevant to nursing as a profession serving humanity. Thus, we can ask the following questions: How will love be considered in nursing education? How can teaching be associated with love?

Teaching From the Heart as an Act of Love

In her recent keynote, Cara (2017) reflected on the nature of both caring and love in nursing. She asked the following questions:

- Are caring and love synonymous?
- Is caring an ingredient for love?
- Are caring and love differentiated by their level of abstraction? For example, caring is more concrete, and love is more abstract [see Figure 4.1].
- Are caring and love distinguished by their level of depth within a relationship [see Figure 4.2]? (pp. 24–28)

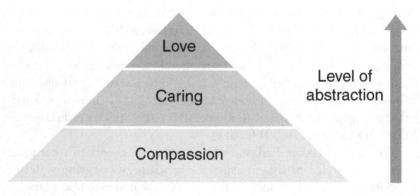

Figure 4.1 Diagram illustrating love and caring according to the level of abstraction.
Source: Adapted from Cara, C. (2017, June). *Rediscovering love, compassion, and caring to alleviate dehumanization.* Keynote speech presented at the 38th International Association for Human Caring Conference, Edmonton, AB, Canada.

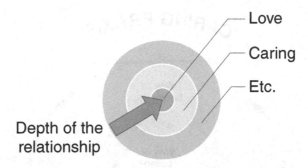

Figure 4.2 Diagram illustrating love and caring according to the level of depth in a relationship.
Source: Adapted from Cara, C. (2017, June). *Rediscovering love, compassion, and caring to alleviate dehumanization.* Keynote speech presented at the 38th International Association for Human Caring Conference, Edmonton, AB, Canada.

Cara (2017) concludes that love as it pertains to the nursing discipline, within clinical, administration, or education domains, is "a virtuous driving force that gives purpose, meaning, and well-being in accomplishing one's life" (p. 35). Love is "virtuous" from having high standards and a moral imperative toward, in our case, students, other nurse educators, as well as the school. Also, love is a "driving force" as it provides the thrust or motivation to care for people, in this instance, our nursing students. It "gives you purpose, meaning, and well-being" as love induces a feeling of fulfillment about caring for students and witnessing their academic success. Finally, finding meaning in one's work makes you feel that you are "accomplishing your life" as well as your professional raison d'être.

In other words, we believe that caring must be anchored on love as the driving force of our Teaching Caring Praxis as nurse educators, allowing us to be in relation with students, in order to contribute to students' harmony, learning, and meaningfulness. Moreover, to be coherent with this perspective, our humanist values (see Chapter 2, Educators' Caring Values, Attitudes, and Behaviors That Contribute to the Humanization of Nursing Education) must transcend it all (see Figure 4.3).

Accordingly, "teaching from the heart as an act of love" may invite nurse educators to see their teaching role as *a virtuous driving force giving purpose, meaning, and well-being in accomplishing oneself as a nurse educator to contribute to students' learning and success.*

At this point, one could ask: How may "teaching from the heart as an act of love" contribute to students' learning, success, and transformation?

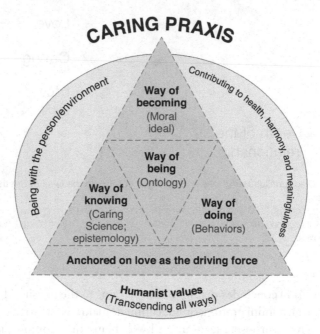

Figure 4.3 Diagram illustrating caring praxis, anchored on love as the driving force.
Source: Adapted from Cara, C. (2017, June). *Rediscovering love, compassion, and caring to alleviate dehumanization.* Keynote speech presented at the 38th International Association for Human Caring Conference, Edmonton, AB, Canada.

TEACHING FROM THE HEART: THE ADDED VALUE FOR STUDENTS AND NURSE EDUCATORS

From our own longtime experience in nursing education, we have perceived that teaching from the heart creates an important difference for both students and nurse educators alike, as being enriching, emancipatory, transformative, and rewarding.

In fact, several authors have acknowledged students' increased learning and growth when nurse educators are teaching from a Human Caring perspective (Beck, 2019; Boykin, Touhy, & Smith, 2011; Flack & Thrall, 2019; Hills & Watson, 2011; Sherman, 2018; Smith, 2019; Whelan, 2017). For example, Sherman (2018) gives various examples of nurse educators' contributions:

> Teaching is reaching into the minds and hearts of students, captivating them with stories, helping them get in touch with their intuitive

selves, and creating the best conditions for learning with respect for varying learning styles, goals, and aspirations. Teaching is bringing out the best in a person, and helping him or her to see his or her potential, while guiding and showing him or her the way through your own example—role modeling the values, attitudes, and behaviors of humanism, professionalism, and excellence in nursing. (p. 73)

In other words, teaching from the heart is being committed to establish trusting relationships with students so that they can feel safe to cocreate knowledge through a respectful dialogue. Therefore, "how" we teach becomes as important as "what" we teach. You may know the class content very well, but being passionate about it is often what will help students to understand its meaningfulness in their future nursing practice. Hence, teaching from the heart contributes to nurture students' questions, reflections, meanings, and learning in order to assist them to reach their fullest potential. As we discussed previously (see Chapter 2, Educators' Caring Values, Attitudes, and Behaviors That Contribute to the Humanization of Nursing Education), to believe in students' potential is an essential humanistic value in nursing education.

Moreover, we invite nurse educators to be inspired by a caring ontology in order to place more emphasis on expanding students' way of "being" and "becoming" rather than focusing mostly on their way of "doing." It implies to be open to a diversity of perceptions, understandings, contexts, and realities. This suggests that nurse educators will consider each student as a unique individual to be accompanied with respect and human dignity. When nurse educators consider each student as being unique, they are, at the same time, teaching them to also consider each patient as a unique person, promoting students' learning in regard to their future caring praxis, as part of our service to humanity.

Lastly, such an approach is also rewarding for nurse educators since they have the opportunity to help students learn to become caring nurses (Beck, 2019; Flack & Thrall, 2019; Hills & Cara, 2019; Hills & Watson, 2011). Indeed, teaching from the heart can bring forth a sense of fulfilment about caring for students and witnessing their academic success and emancipation as they familiarize to share their voice, to engage in their reflective practice, to express their apprehensions and interrogations in order to reach their professional goals and learn to eventually transform healthcare and humanize nursing practice. From our own experience, these kinds of rewards are what give meaning to one's own practice as nurse educators.

TIME OUT FOR REFLECTION

We invite you to write your reflection in a journal in order to link the preceding theoretical segment with your personal teaching/learning experiences.

Think about a time when you were in a situation where it felt that you were "teaching from the heart," and ask yourself these questions:

- What were the characteristics reflecting teaching from the heart?
- What was your lived experience like?
- What specific pedagogical activities were involved in this experience?
- What were the advantages for your students' learning?
- What were the advantages for your relationships with your students?
- What were the advantages for your own teaching/learning practice?

TEACHING FROM THE HEART: EXAMPLES OF SOME PEDAGOGICAL ACTIVITIES

Table 4.1 contains some examples of various pedagogical activities that can assist nurse educators to be "teaching from the heart."

Table 4.1 Example of Pedagogical Activities Related to Teaching From the Heart

Pedagogical Activities	Authors
Centering before going into the classroom	Vitali (2019) Watson (2018b)
Honoring students' human dignity and experiences	Cara and Hills (2018) Hills and Cara (2019) Hills and Watson (2011) Vitali (2019) (See also Chapter 2, Educators' Caring Values, Attitudes, and Behaviors That Contribute to the Humanization of Nursing Education)
Considering both students and nurse educators as learners	Cara and Hills (2018) Vitali (2019) Watson (2018a) (See also Chapter 5, Seeking Teaching/Learning Caring Relationships With Students)

(continued)

Table 4.1 Example of Pedagogical Activities Related to Teaching From the Heart *(Continued)*

Pedagogical Activities	Authors
Providing a caring and safe environment in the classroom	Cara et al. (2016) Cara and Hills (2018) Rockwood Lane and Samuels (2011) Vitali (2019)
Being guided by Teaching Caritas Processes	See Chapter 6, Caritas Processes and Caritas Literacy as a Teaching Guide for Enlightened Nurse Educators
Considering teaching as a relational human process to cocreate knowledge	Cara and Girard (2013) Cara and Hills (2018) Hills and Cara (2019) (See also Chapter 5, Seeking Teaching/Learning Caring Relationships With Students)
Choosing "power with" rather than "power over"	Hills and Cara (2019) Hills and Watson (2011) (See also Chapter 3, Emancipatory Contributions to Humanize Nursing Education)

As developed in Chapter 6, Caritas Processes and Caritas Literacy as a Teaching Guide for Enlightened Nurse Educators, the seventh Teaching Caritas Process, *Engaging in transpersonal teaching and learning within context of caring student–educator relationship; staying within the student's frame of reference-shift toward coaching model for expanded learning,* is particularly significant to nurse educators in their teaching practice. For Watson (2008), teaching necessitates a genuine and caring relationship based on trust, respecting each person as a whole human being. The seventh Teaching Caritas Process invites nurse educators to be in sync with students' rhythm of learning, as a reminder that each student's learning experience is unique. Said differently, we are convinced that being in sync with students' rhythm can make a difference in their learning as they can better grasp and understand knowledge related to nursing practice.

We believe that these activities can assist nurse educators to teach from the heart. Nonetheless, these examples are not the only ways to teach from the heart, but they are offered rather as suggestions to begin this process.

PRAGMATIC SEGMENT
TEACHING FROM THE HEART

Nancy J. Vitali, DCS, MS, RN

Words not supported by the energy of personal experiences have much less power than words grounded in personal experience that possess the energy of love and caring.

—Watson, 2008, p. 258

A Profound Experience of Love

It was a profound experience of love and caring that guided my teaching partner, Dr. Lisa Gerow, and myself to reconsider our teaching approach in our undergraduate psychiatric mental health nursing course. Our students were reticent to discuss and ask questions in our class, leaving us frustrated and concerned as to whether or not they were learning. We wondered that perhaps they were intimidated or felt stigmatized by the subject matter, but we had no ready solutions for sparking their engagement in the course.

In November 2006, we traveled to Oklahoma City to participate in a lectureship day that Oklahoma State University sponsored. The speaker was Dr. Jean Watson. That day marked the beginning of a 12-year Caritas journey into Human Caring and healing, compassion, wisdom, and love, which culminated in a doctoral degree in Caring Science from the Watson Caring Science Institute, and it was graced with loving, caring encounters with other caring faculty and nurses in clinical practice.

Dr. Watson explicated her theory as she applied it to nursing education. She described caring via the Chinese symbol for "passage to the heart" (Jean Watson, Margaret Brock Lectureship, November 3, 2006). She elucidated Levinas' "ethics of face" and encouraged us to be aware of and open to "connecting with the infinite field of universal Love in the moment" when interacting with our students (Watson, 2008). She also cited the importance of multiple ways of knowing in planning courses (Carper, 1978; Chinn & Kramer, 2015). Besides, we were reminded of Nightingale's premise that nursing is a calling and we should approach our students with respect and reverence for the journey that each student had embarked upon. We took all this in with new attention, excitement, and focus.

Despite the impact of the eloquence, scholarship, and inspiration that flowed from Dr. Watson's teachings, what really motivated us to change was her sharing her story of a personal tragedy near the end of the day. Her conscious act of opening her heart to an audience of over 200 strangers motivated and inspired us to open our hearts to our students by sharing the challenges and vulnerabilities of mental illnesses in our own families via a family diagram activity on the opening day of class each semester. We also began to use different pedagogical approaches to the course we taught, including music videos and lyrics as poetry, storytelling, and role-playing mental health scenarios. Beginning each class with popular music and discussion of the visual, musical, and poetic aspects of videos, as they related to specific mental illnesses and recovery/healing, engaged the students and decreased their fear of sharing in public. Our classes became more interactive and vibrant, and students remarked on the caring and concern we showed toward them as well as the rich learning experiences, both informally and on our course evaluations.

HeartMath and Beyond
As the journey continued, a centering, heart-focused meditation called HeartMath® Quick Coherence (HeartMath, n.d.) was added to each class and before each exam. Although quantitative studies were not conducted, qualitative feedback from the students who used it was positive, and as the only teacher of HeartMath in the program, I received many thanks over the 10 years it was taught from students who benefited from it.

A class focusing on culture as a foundation for holistic health was included, in which each student was asked to bring an object that represented a culture they were part of. Describing their cultural connections honored each person's subjective experience. This activity was conducted in a circle, using the Native American tradition of the talking stick to highlight the primacy of listening in mental health nursing. A teaching about indigenous cultures' spiritual belief in the interrelatedness of all beings was included in the introduction to the activity. The students were attentive and focused during the sharing and were often amazed at the array of beautiful clothing, artifacts, books, heartfelt stories, songs, and photos of loved ones from the varied cultures and locations represented by classmates from Africa to rural Oklahoma. This activity undoubtedly served to create a bridge of understanding and respect across the diverse ethnicities and locales of the students, while providing valuable cross-cultural understanding. This understanding and deep connection was experienced rather than taught, as students learned Human Caring through heart connections to one another as they listened to one another's stories.

The Gifts of Caring Teachers

The most recent chapter in my journey, in regard to "teaching from the heart," involved interviewing 10 experienced nursing teachers from the United States and Canada to honor their stories and record their experiences of this phenomenon, as part of my doctoral dissertation research (Vitali, 2017). It was not expected that their stories would match mine and Dr. Gerow's, and they did not. All 10 teachers' stories revealed six themes associated with teaching from a heart-centered rather than strictly a knowledge and skills acquisition approach:

- It's a hard job
- Knowing and living caring
- Embracing vulnerability
- Learning and growing together
- Being in right relationship
- Experiencing spiritual transformation (Vitali, 2017, p. 153)

Here, these themes are exemplified from the participants' stories. I will refer to these teachers by the pseudonyms used in my research. The students are not named.

Several teachers described interactions with students who were struggling in nursing school for either personal or academic reasons. For them, teaching from the heart meant that they were kind, attentive, and supportive of students. For example, Annie explored what made a student want to be in healthcare when it was certain that the student was not going to succeed in nursing. On discovering that his desire was to care for others, Annie assisted the student to find a suitable, less physically invasive discipline other than nursing. Annie's story especially reflects the themes "knowing and living caring" and "learning and growing together" because of her statement that she walked arm-in-arm with students as they learned together (Vitali, 2017, p. 153).

Two teachers in this study worked hard to develop trusting/caring relationships with students who were afraid of them. Simone did this by seeking mentoring at the university where she teaches as well as completing a nurse coach program focusing on Caring Science, which subsequently shifted her entire approach to teaching from focusing on sociopolitical aspects of nursing to one emphasizing Human Caring. Regarding the change this has brought about in the classroom, Simone shared that she serves tea to her students whenever she can and that student evaluations no longer reflect a lack of connection with their needs. Simone's story particularly related to the themes "embracing vulnerability" and "being in right relationship" (Vitali, 2017, p. 153).

For her part, Grace let a student know that her beliefs were honored and welcomed when the student struggled with practices such as meditation because of religious reasons. Grace's story notably illustrated the theme "embracing vulnerability" (Vitali, 2017, p. 153). She asserted, "I learned that whenever I feel angst, that if I can embrace that as a teachable moment, and turn this situation where both I and the student have the opportunity to learn and grow, that will absolutely transform our relationship" (Vitali, 2017, p. 140). Grace went on to describe the feelings of fear and vulnerability at that moment of angst between herself and a student. She shared the many activities she uses to maintain balance, such as meditation, Pilates, time with a pet, and consulting a Shaman.

Another teacher, Shamus, created healing environments so that students could survive a capstone experience in a Central American country. She shared a story of traveling a great distance by bus to console a student who was homesick and, on another occasion, of finding foods a student could eat when indigenous foods were not tolerated. Her story related especially to the theme "It's a hard job" (Vitali, 2017, p. 153). Regarding difficult times in foreign countries, she explained, "Oh, wow. Those are very complex. And you vacillate from being a teacher, to a mentor, to a mom . . . and you have to be their rock. I've done it enough now, that I know the pattern that occurs with students, so I'm better prepared to meet their needs" (Vitali, 2017, p. 132).

Lark coached a student through his first encounter with death and dying, when he was so overwhelmed by emotion that he could not function. She spent 30 minutes with this young man away from the patient room, sharing her first experience with death, so that he could be present to the pain and suffering of the family of the dying patient.

Another teacher, Rumi, received a call from a student who was crying, having forgotten to take an exam because her significant other was in the ICU. Being concerned, Rumi simply inquired if the student had eaten anything that day. This teacher also broke a rule of the nursing school where she taught, allowing the student to take the missed exam, and on graduation day, the student sent her a plant with a note telling her, "You are why I am graduating on Friday. I just wanted to say, 'Thanks'" (Vitali, 2017, p. 151).

Annie honored mysterious, unexplainable events and exemplified the theme "experiencing a spiritual transformation" by telling the story of a student who cared with enormous presence and tenderness for a dying patient and shared in her miraculous recovery (Vitali, 2017). Annie explained, "And every time I went to check on them, my soul cried, because she was in there—she had the blinds open, sunlight streaming in; she was playing music; she was singing to the patient" (Vitali, 2017, p. 152).

For Rumi and Annie, experiencing a spiritual transformation was central to their experiences as nurse educators. Rumi asserted that she saw each student as a precious crystal bead that reflected the light of every other crystal bead (soul). This nurse educator stated, "Sometimes we have to listen to our heart and see that person, that unique individual and respond to that, but it can be hard. It is a difficult balance" (Vitali, 2017, p. 151).

Conclusion

The experiences of participants of this qualitative study and from my own lived experience as a faculty member, appear to show that "teaching from the heart" can facilitate students' learning to be caring nurses. One can reasonably expect that those students who have been shown such caring and kindness will in turn extend that experience to others in their lives as nurses.

In summary, teaching from the heart is not formulaic. It is as individualistic as the nurse educators who embrace it. A key element from the first Caritas Process (Watson, 2008) is that loving-kindness and equanimity are also directed toward nurse educators so that the life-giving cycle is complete, making this sacred path of teaching and learning, with those who are entering the discipline, a sustainable and joyful one.

CONCLUSION

This chapter intended to raise nurse educators' consciousness about the importance to be teaching from the heart and its contribution to humanize nursing education as well as its added value to facilitate students' learning. Lastly, Vitali's Pragmatic Segment exemplified clearly the content of this chapter.

Watson eloquently claims that love in nursing education is:

love of nursing, love of learning, love of diversity, love of challenge of ideas, love of knowledge, and love of sharing knowledge with kindness and patience, in ways that inspire, invite, and create safe space to listen, to ask questions, to disagree, and to evolve together. Be open to hear what students (and patients) have to teach you. You as the *faculty* become *expert learner* along with your students. (Watson, 2018a, p. 189)

In closing, as nurse educators, we need to recognize that we can, for better or for worse, subjugate or empower our students. Hence, teaching from the heart corresponds to a humanistic way to empower students. Teaching from the heart can become an act of caring, an act of love. We believe that such an act of love not only gives meaning to nurse educators' daily teaching practice, a primary raison d'être to pursue one's caring praxis within nursing education, but it contributes to making a difference in students' lives. Such a difference in students' learning journey can not only inspire them to learn new knowledge, but it can also be pivotal in whether or not they will become future caring nurses, future empowered caring leaders, and future caring social activists, concerned in advancing healthcare humanization for all, therefore, also making a difference in the life and health of patients, families, communities, and populations of the world.

REFERENCES

Beck, M. D. (2019). Fostering metamorphosis through caring literacy in an RN-to-BSN program. In W. Rosa, S. Horton-Deutsch, & J. Watson (Eds.), *A handbook for Caring Science: Expanding the paradigm* (pp. 257–275). New York, NY: Springer Publishing Company.

Benner, P., Sutphen, M., Leonard, V., & Day, L. (2010). *Educating nurses: A call for radical transformation.* San Francisco, CA: Jossey-Bass.

Boykin, A., & Schoenhofer, S. (2013). Caring in nursing: Analysis of extant theory. In M. C. Smith, M. C. Turkel, & Z. Robinson Wolf (Eds.), *Caring in nursing classics: An essential resource* (pp. 33–42). New York, NY: Springer Publishing Company.

Boykin, A., Touhy, T. A., & Smith, M. C. (2011). Evolution of a caring-based college of nursing. In M. Hills, & J. Watson (Eds.), *Creating a Caring Science curriculum: An emancipatory pedagogy for nursing* (pp. 157–184). New York, NY: Springer Publishing Company.

Cara, C. (2017, June). *Rediscovering love, compassion, and caring to alleviate dehumanization.* Keynote speech presented at the 38th International Association for Human Caring Conference, Edmonton, AB, Canada.

Cara, C., Gauvin-Lepage, J., Lefebvre, H., Létourneau, D., Alderson, M., Larue, C., . . . Mathieu, C. (2016). Le Modèle humaniste des soins infirmiers—UdeM: perspective novatrice et pragmatique. *Recherche en soins infirmiers, 125*, 20–31. doi:10.3917/rsi.125.0020

Cara, C., & Girard, F. (2013, May). *The humanist model of nursing care: A driving force for nursing education.* Poster session presented at the 34th International Association for Human Caring Conference, Lake Buena Vista, FL.

Cara, C., & Hills, M. (2018, May). *The added value of Caring Science: Its contributions to humanize nursing education.* Oral presentation at the Canadian Association of Schools in Nursing Conference, Montreal, QC, Canada.

Carper, B. A. (1978). Fundamental patterns of knowing in nursing. *Advances in Nursing Science, 1*, 13–23. doi:10.1097/00012272-197810000-00004

Chinn, P., & Kramer, M. (2015). *Knowledge development in nursing: Theory and process* (9th ed.). St. Louis, MO: Elsevier.

Fitzgerald, L. (1998). Is it possible for caring to be an expression of human agape in the 21st century? *International Journal for Human Caring, 2*(3), 32–39. doi:10.20467/1091-5710.2.3.32

Flack, L. L., & Thrall, D. (2019). Developing values and philosophies of being. In W. Rosa, S. Horton-Deutsch, & J. Watson (Eds.), *A handbook for Caring Science: Expanding the paradigm* (pp. 243–256). New York, NY: Springer Publishing Company.

Goldin, M. (2016). Empathic and unselfish: Redefining nurse caring as love in action. In W. Rosa (Ed.), *Nurses as leaders: Evolutionary visions of leadership* (pp. 279–291). New York, NY: Springer Publishing Company.

Goldin, M. (2017). *Nursing as love: A hermeneutical phenomenological study of the creative thought within nursing* (Unpublished doctoral dissertation). Watson Caring Science Institute, Boulder, CO.

Goldin, M. (2019). Nursing as love: A hermeneutical phenomenological study of the creative thought within nursing. In W. Rosa, S. Horton-Deutsch, & J. Watson (Eds.), *A handbook for Caring Science: Expanding the paradigm* (pp. 433–446). New York, NY: Springer Publishing Company.

HeartMath. (n.d.). *Quick Coherence® Technique*. Retrieved from https://www .heartmath.com/quick-coherence-technique

Hills, M., & Cara, C. (2019). Curriculum development processes and pedagogical practices for advancing Caring Science literacy. In W. Rosa, S. Horton-Deutsch, & J. Watson (Eds.), *A handbook for Caring Science: Expanding the paradigm* (pp. 197–210). New York, NY: Springer Publishing Company.

Hills, M., & Watson, J. (2011). *Creating a Caring Science curriculum: An emancipatory pedagogy for nursing*. New York, NY: Springer Publishing Company.

Hunt, D. D. (2018). *The new nurse educator: Mastering academe* (2nd ed.). New York, NY: Springer Publishing Company.

Palmer, J. P. (1997). The heart of a teacher identity and integrity in teaching. *Change: The Magazine of Higher Learning, 29*(6), 14–21. doi:10.1080/00091389709602343

Rockwood Lane, M., & Samuels, M. (2011). Introduction to caring as a pedagogical approach to nursing education. In M. Hills & J. Watson (Eds.), *Creating a Caring Science curriculum: An emancipatory pedagogy for nursing* (pp. 217–244). New York, NY: Springer Publishing Company.

Sherman, D. (2018). Reflections about scholarship, teaching, and service: The expectations of academic nursing. In D. D. Hunt (Ed.), *The new nurse educator: Mastering academe* (2nd ed., pp. 71–76). New York, NY: Springer Publishing Company.

Smith, M. C. (2019). Advancing Caring Science through the missions of teaching, research/scholarship, practice, and service. In W. Rosa, S. Horton-Deutsch, & J. Watson (Eds.), *A handbook for Caring Science: Expanding the paradigm* (pp. 285–301). New York, NY: Springer Publishing Company.

Stickley, T., & Freshwater, D. (2002). The art of loving and the therapeutic relationship. *Nursing Inquiry, 9*(4), 250–256. doi:10.1046/j.1440-1800.2002.00155.x

Swanson, K. M. (2013). What is known about caring in nursing science: A literary meta-analysis. In M. C. Smith, M. C. Turkel, & Z. R. Wolf (dir.) (Eds.), *Caring in nursing classics: An essential resource* (pp. 59–102). New York, NY: Springer Publishing Company.

Thorkildsen, K. M., Eriksson, K., & Raholm, M.-B. (2013). The substance of love when encountering suffering: An interpretive research synthesis with an abductive approach. *Scandinavian Journal of Caring Science, 27*, 449–459. doi:10.1111/j.1471-6712.2012.01038.x

Thorkildsen, K. M., Eriksson, K., & Raholm, M.-B. (2015). The core of love when caring for patients suffering from addiction. *Scandinavian Journal of Caring Science, 29*, 353–360. doi:10.1111/scs.12171

Vitali, N. (2017). *Nursing faculty experience of teaching from the heart* (Unpublished doctoral dissertation). Watson Caring Science Institute, Boulder, CO.

Vitali, N. (2019). Teaching from the heart. In W. Rosa, S. Horton-Deutsch, & J. Watson (Eds.), *A handbook for Caring Science: Expanding the paradigm* (pp. 225–241). New York, NY: Springer Publishing Company.

Watson, J. (2006, November). *Margaret Brock lectureship*. Oklahoma City: Oklahoma State University.

Watson, J. (2008). *Nursing: The philosophy and science of caring* (revised ed.). Boulder: University Press of Colorado.

Watson, J. (2017). Global Human Caring for a sustainable world. In W. Rosa (Ed.), *A new era in global health: Nursing and the United Nations 2030 Agenda for sustainable development* (pp. 223–241). New York, NY: Springer Publishing Company.

Watson, J. (2018a). Reflection on teaching and sustaining Human Caring. In D. D. Hunt (Ed.), *The new nurse educator: Mastering academe* (2nd ed., pp. 189–194). New York, NY: Springer Publishing Company.

Watson, J. (2018b). *Unitary Caring Science: The philosophy and praxis of nursing*. Louisville: University of Colorado Press.

Whelan, J. (2017). The Caring Science imperative: A hallmark in nursing education. In S. Lee, P. Palmieri, & J. Watson (Eds.), *Global advances in Human Caring literacy* (pp. 33–42). New York, NY: Springer Publishing Company.

5

Seeking Teaching/Learning Caring Relationships With Students

We believe that learning actually occurs at the juncture of the authentic caring relationship that is created and lived by the teacher and students and the knowledge that they cocreate. Learning is a dynamic lived human experience. An emancipatory relational pedagogy aims to create a relationship between teacher, learner, and knowledge that is based on a carefully edified thoughtfulness that attends to people's lived experiences and the meanings they create from those experiences. This notion of lived experience and its inherent concept of meaning making are at the heart of understanding emancipatory relational pedagogies.
—Hills and Watson, 2011, p. 62

LEARNING INTENTIONS

- Reflect on how a Human Caring perspective may inform nurse educators as to how to develop relationships with their students.
- Sensitize nurse educators about the importance of the relational nature of their work with students.
- Appreciate how teaching/learning caring relationships contribute to students' learning and knowledge cocreation and to humanizing nursing education.
- Understand, from a student's perspective, how a teaching/learning caring relationship can promote learning and success.

INTRODUCTION

Several authors recognize the importance of the student–educator rela-tionship when teaching nursing. However, when describing this important phenomenon in the nursing education realm, different authors use different constructs, sometimes interchangeably (see Table 5.1).

Of all the different terms used in the nursing literature, the expression *student–teacher relationship* is predominant. In order to explicate the influence that a caring ontology has on the relationship, we begin this chapter by revis-iting the work of Watson. We then introduce the construct *teaching/learning caring relationship* to better illustrate that within the caring relationship, both the educator and the student are teaching and learning.

This chapter aims to elucidate how nurse educators can create and sustain teaching/learning caring relationships with students in order to

Table 5.1 **Different Constructs Used in the Nursing Literature**

Constructs Used	Authors
Student–teacher relationship	Beck (2001); Bevis and Watson (1989, 2000); Boykin, Touhy, and Smith (2011); Cara et al. (2016); Cara and Hills (2018); Chan, Tong, and Henderson (2017); Froneman, Du Plessis, and Koen (2016); Gillespie (2005); Hills and Cara (2019); Hills and Watson (2011); Labrague, McEnroe-Petitte, Papathanasiou, Edet, and Arulappa (2015); Ray (2010); Sitzman and Watson (2017); Smith and Crowe (2017); Touhy and Boykin (2008); Watson (2000); Whelan (2017)
Student–teacher interaction	Beck (2001); Bevis and Watson (1989, 2000); Labrague et al. (2015); Sitzman (2007)
Student–teacher connection	Beck (2001); Gillespie (2005); Grams, Kosowsky, and Wilson (1997)
Student–teacher connectedness	Labrague et al. (2015); Miller, Haber, and Byrne (1990); Sitzman (2007)
Student–teacher interconnectedness	Sitzman (2007)
Student–teacher transactions	Bevis and Watson (1989, 2000)
Student–teacher encounter	Halldorsdottir (1990)

improve students' learning of caring practices and simultaneously cocreate knowledge. Such an approach contributes to humanizing nursing education. With that in mind, this chapter is intended to sensitize nurse educators about the importance of the relational nature of their work with students and to coach them on how to develop and maintain a teaching/learning caring relationship with their students.

RELATIONAL NATURE OF NURSE EDUCATORS' WORK

The relational nature of nurse educators' work with students is crucial; therefore, it is essential to discuss how to develop and maintain a *teaching/ learning caring relationship* with students. Such a relationship calls for nurse educators to transcend the mere objective assessment and evaluation of students by showing concern for their deep subjective understanding and meaning of their own learning experience.

By underscoring an ontology of caring within nursing education, the nurse educator's role becomes a relational human process. Such perspective implies, for nurse educators, to "be with" students, honoring their beliefs, perceptions, meanings, "skillfulness" (Benner, 2005), as well as their learning of relevant knowledge for their future caring practice with patients, families, and communities. Consequently, from such a perspective, nursing students cannot be considered as mere passive, docile, or obedient receptacles to be filled up with the content selected by nurse educators to be learned. Rather, nursing students must be considered as active, dynamic, participating cocreators of knowledge and meanings.

An ontology of caring within nursing education also recognizes the significance of the student–educator relationship as being essential for students' learning to occur and flourish. Several authors also claim that the student–educator relationship is critical to enhancing students' learning (Boykin, Touhy, & Smith, 2011; Cara et al., 2016; Cara & Hills, 2018; Chan, Tong, & Henderson, 2017; Froneman, Du Plessis, & Koen, 2016; Hills & Cara, 2019; Hills & Watson, 2011; Labrague, McEnroe-Petitte, Papathanasiou, Edet, & Arulappa, 2015; Noddings, 2012, 2013; Smith & Crowe, 2017; Whelan, 2017).

WATSON'S WORK REVISITED

The transpersonal caring relationship is the cornerstone of Watson's *Human Caring Science*. From this perspective, the transpersonal caring relationship should be as meaningful to nurse educators as it is to clinical nurses. Before describing this concept as it relates to education, it is important to understand its meaning in a nurse–patient relationship.

Watson's Nurse–Patient Transpersonal Caring Relationship

The transpersonal caring relationship is explained by Watson (2012) as follows:

> [It] begins when the nurse enters into the life space or phenomenal field of another person, is able to detect the other person's condition of being (spirit, soul), feels this condition within him- or her-self, and responds to the condition in such a way that the recipient has a release of subjective feelings and thoughts he or she had been longing to release. As such, there is an intersubjective flow between the nurse and patient. As feelings, thoughts, and energies that are less harmonious with either person's self are released, they become replaced by other feelings, thoughts, and energies that are more harmonious with one's self and are kinder toward and more mindful of the well-being of each person and ultimately for humankind. (p. 75)

In other words, a transpersonal caring relationship allows the nurse to achieve a deeper connection with the person in order to promote the other's well-being, healing, harmony, and empowerment. Moreover, Watson's (2018) transpersonal caring relationship is linked to an ontology of being and becoming, acknowledging an authentic spiritual presence in the moment as well as the highest level of consciousness, both of which are recommended for healing to occur.

Watson (1999) specifies that the term "transpersonal," in describing a caring relationship, means going beyond one's own ego and not denying or objectifying the person (Watson, 1999). Indeed, a *transpersonal caring relationship* is fundamentally guided by an ethic, a moral ideal to protect, enhance, and preserve human dignity (Watson, 2018). "A transpersonal caring relationship connotes a special kind of human care relationship—a connection/union with another person, a high regard for the whole person and their being-in-the-world. Caring, in this sense, is viewed as the moral ideal of nursing where there is the utmost concern for human dignity and preservation of humanity" (Watson, 2012, p. 75).

Student–Educator Transpersonal Caring Relationship

By introducing the transpersonal caring relationship into nursing education, nurse educators create a *student–educator transpersonal caring relationship* with their students. If the ultimate goal of a transpersonal caring relationship is to protect, enhance, and preserve a person's human dignity, wholeness, and inner harmony, then, in the context of nursing education, the ultimate goal of a student–educator *transpersonal caring relationship* would be to protect, enhance, and preserve students' human dignity, integrative learning, and inner harmony.

According to Watson (2012), transpersonal caring relationships have certain prerequisites. The adaptation of these prerequisites for nursing education is detailed in Table 5.2.

Table 5.2 **Watson's Prerequisites Adapted for Nurse Education**

Clinical Standpoint	Educational Standpoint
1. A moral commitment to protect and enhance human dignity, wherein a person is allowed to determine his or her own meaning.	1. The nurse educator's moral commitment to protect and enhance the student's learning and human dignity, wherein the student is allowed to determine his or her own meanings and learning within the nursing program.
2. The nurse's intent and will to affirm the subjective, spiritual significance of the person.	2. The nurse educator's intent and will to affirm the subjective, spiritual significance of the student.
3. The nurse's ability to realize and accurately detect feelings and the inner condition of another. To seek "to see" and connect spirit-to-spirit with the other, even in the moment. This can occur through authentic presence, being open, intentional and mindful with actions, words, behaviors, cognition, body language, feelings, thought, senses, intuition, and so on.	3. The nurse educator's ability to realize and accurately detect feelings pertaining to the student's learning. To seek "to see" and connect spirit-to-spirit with the student, even in the teaching/learning moment. This can occur through authentic presence, being open, intentional and mindful with pedagogical strategies, actions, words, behaviors, cognition, body language, feelings, thought, senses, intuition, and so on.
4. The ability of the nurse to assess and realize another's condition of being-in-the-world and to feel a human-to-human connection with another.	4. The ability of the nurse educator to assess and realize the student's condition of being-in-the-world within the nursing program and the nursing profession and to feel a human-to-human connection with the student.

(continued)

Table 5.2 Watson's Prerequisites Adapted for Nurse Education
(Continued)

Clinical Standpoint	Educational Standpoint
5. The nurse's own life history (collective past) and previous experiences, culture, background, and opportunities of having lived through or experienced one's own feelings and various human conditions and of having imagined others' feelings and sufferings from various human conditions.	5. The nurse educator's own life history (collective past) and previous pedagogical experiences, teaching culture, background, and opportunities of having lived through or experienced one's own feelings and various apprenticeship conditions and of having imagined the students' feelings and academic difficulties and sufferings from various learning conditions.

Source: Adapted from Watson, J. (2012). *Human Caring Science: A theory of nursing* (p. 76). Sudbury, MA: Jones & Bartlett Learning.

In nursing education, nurse educators and students develop mutuality within their relationship. Furthermore, in a student–educator caring moment, this mutuality can contribute to the student's learning of becoming a caring nurse and can foster a sense of well-being within the nursing program. Nurse educators' authentic presence and entering into and staying within students' frame of reference are required to help students' professional growth and emancipation. Such a presence will assist nurse educators to consider students' learning rhythm in order to help them grasp and integrate knowledge as well as to find meaning in relevant caring–healing practices in nursing. Emancipation can thereby be experienced more profoundly within these *student–educator transpersonal caring relationships* (see Figure 5.1).

In her work, Watson (2012) also uses the expression "art of transpersonal caring" (p. 80). She clarifies that transpersonal caring corresponds to the nurse being able to alleviate all separation with the other, illustrating a real reciprocity with the person, and connecting deeply with compassion and concern on a level that transcends the physical toward a greater and more profound meaning. With that in mind, the *student–educator transpersonal caring relationship* may contribute to help students develop a higher/deeper consciousness and harmony and, more specifically, caring–healing praxis.

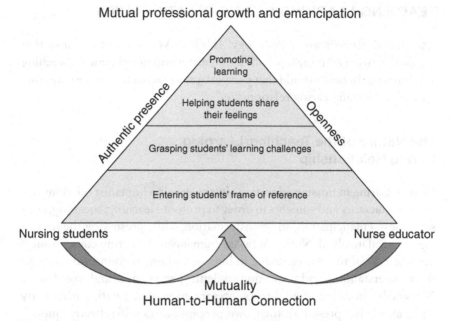

Figure 5.1 Student–teacher transpersonal caring relationship diagram.

TIME OUT FOR REFLECTION

You can write your reflection in a journal in order to link the preceding theoretical segment with your personal *student–educator transpersonal caring relationship* developed with your students.

Think about a situation where you felt that you could have better helped and supported one of your students facing a challenge, and then ask yourself the following questions:

- Who was involved?
- What was your lived experience?
- How did you feel?
- What were you telling yourself at the time?
- What were the impacts for your student? And for your teaching practice?
- How could you have established a *student–educator transpersonal caring relationship*?
- How could this *student–educator transpersonal caring relationship* have helped your student's challenge? Your student's professional growth?
- How could this *student–educator transpersonal caring relationship* have helped your own professional growth?

TEACHING/LEARNING CARING RELATIONSHIPS

"Relational Emancipatory Pedagogy" (Hills & Watson, 2011) claims that within the caring relationship, both the educator and the student are teaching and learning. In order to add that perspective, we have chosen the construct "teaching/learning caring relationship."

The Nature of the Teaching/Learning Caring Relationship

Human Caring in nursing education aims to develop humanist relationships among educators and students in order to promote learning, meaning, consciousness, emancipation, and transformation, while preserving the human dignity of all involved. Nurse educators' humanism and caring consciousness become crucial to their engaging in human-to-human connections and to their understanding and respecting students' perspectives and worldviews. Nurse educators are invited to be present to students with authenticity while also being present to their own perceptions (a self-reflective mode). Consequently, a caring relationship underlines the uniqueness of all persons, be they nurse educators or students, as well as the mutuality, trust, and equity within the educator–student relationship. Indeed, a *teaching/learning caring relationship* must be respectful, authentic, humanist, and based on equity, trust, and safety (see Figure 5.2). As outlined in Chapter 2, Educators' Caring Values, Attitudes, and Behaviors That Contribute to the Humanization of Nursing Education, caring values and attitudes are relevant elements to a caring relationship.

In this type of relationship, both nurse educators and students join in a mutual search for meaning and wholeness as well as for the cocreation of knowledge within a safe environment. In other words, the perspective of Relational Emancipatory Pedagogy acknowledges that, in the relationship, both are learners and both are teachers. Consequently, teaching/learning caring relationships can assist nurse educators to cocreate knowledge that is meaningful to students' caring practice with patients.

For Hills and Watson (2011), this kind of relationship is a prerequisite for the cocreation of knowledge. They claim

> learning occurs at the juncture or intersection when the teacher and students are in a caring relationship and are cocreating knowledge. They are engaged in a process of transformational learning in which they cocreate knowledge through the complex caring relational process: relation with subject matter; relation with own ideas and personal

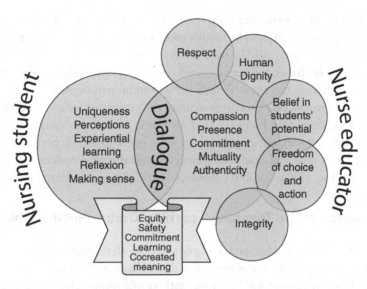

Figure 5.2 Diagram illustrating the teaching/learning caring relationship.

meaning; through relation with peers / classmates / social-political dynamics; and through caring student-teacher relationship among other relational dynamics of inner subjective experiences. (p. 53)

When nurse educators, within their *teaching/learning caring relationship* with students, inspire and support their students to discuss caring values, caring attitudes, and caring behaviors as well as how they contribute to alleviate patients' and families' suffering, they promote the students' learning of what it means to be/become a caring nurse. We contend that such a teaching perspective contributes to humanizing nursing education. It should be the educators' moral imperative to develop a *teaching/learning caring relationship* with students. Nurse educators nurturing caring relationships among students is critical as their learning of the profession depends on it. "From an educator's perspective, helping students develop caring literacy is a moral imperative because caring is the very essence of nursing. How we, as educators, instill and nurture caring among students is vital—through respect for humanity, dignity, and body/mind/spirit holism" (Whelan, 2017, p. 40).

Depth of the Teaching/Learning Caring Relationship

We believe that these *student–teacher caring relationships* correspond to the highest level of relationships as the "life-giving" or "biogenic" mode of being with another person (Halldorsdottir, 1991, 2013). As claimed by Halldorsdottir, this mode involves a true presence as well as an interconnectedness, allowing the other person to expand her or his consciousness with spiritual freedom. Halldorsdottir (1991, 2013) asserts that by creating such relationships based on respect, compassion, openness, and receptivity, such a life-giving mode of being enhances the person's well-being and human dignity.

In nursing education, we propose using the expression "teaching/learning-giving/receiving" (see Figure 5.3). This mode of being is congruent with the *teaching/learning caring relationship* as it involves a true presence from nurse educators as well as an interconnectedness allowing students to expand their learning, meanings, and consciousness along with spiritual freedom.

Relevance of the Teaching/Learning Caring Relationship

In the clinical realm, Human Caring has to do with relationships, where the main goal is improving the person's health and healing. Within the education realm, Human Caring still has to do with relationships, those of the nurse educators and students, but here, the foremost purpose of this relationship is students' learning. At the same time, one can wonder why relationships are so vital to teaching nursing as well as to promoting students' academic learning, professional growth, and even resilience.

In their exploratory qualitative study with 40 nursing auxiliary students from a private institution in South Africa, Froneman et al. (2016) studied the "educator–student relationships" and how they strengthen students' resilience. They believe that "strengthening students' resilience from the beginning of their nursing career through a positive and supportive educator–student relationship can improve their well-being as well as uplift the quality of education, thereby improving the quality of patient care delivered" (p. 2). Their results reveal, among other things, that in order to have an effective educator–student relationship, the teaching/learning environment must be based on mutual respect and openness, that the interaction must be constructive and always acknowledge students' human rights, and that both educators and students must manifest specific qualities (Froneman et al., 2016). For example, students considered the following qualities as being important for the educators to display: "loving, caring, respectful, responsible, moral, patient, open to new ideas, motivated, willingness to go 'the extra mile,' and punctual" (Froneman et al., 2016, p. 6). Despite the fact that this study is limited to a private institution in a semiurban area of South Africa, that it did not explore the *teaching/learning caring relationship* specifically, and that it did not consider the teachers' perspective, the results do contribute to an understanding of the added value of student–educator relationships.

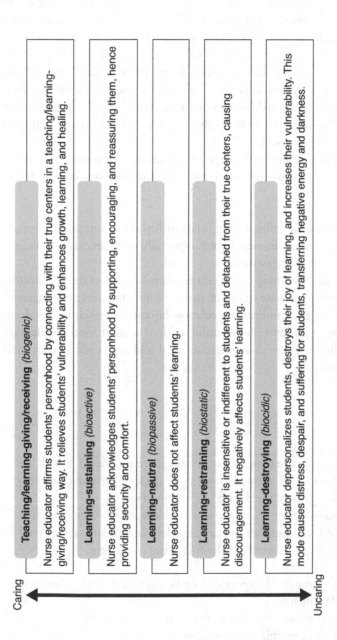

Figure 5.3 Adaptation for nursing education of Halldorsdottir's modes of being.

Source: Adapted from Halldorsdottir, S. (2013). Five basic modes of being with another. In M. C. Smith, M. C. Turkel, & Z.R. Wolf (Eds.), *Caring in nursing classics: An essential resource* (pp. 201–210). New York, NY: Springer Publishing Company.

From a nurse educators' perspective, Smith and Crowe (2017) conducted a qualitative descriptive study with 10 nurse educators teaching online classes in the United States. Their findings pinpoint that nurse educators consider their relationships with their students as an essential part of their teaching to assist students with learning difficulties and promote students' engagement to their global learning. These researchers concluded that nursing teachers have to know their students in order to understand their needs and that they have to be responsive to those needs to help them build relationships. Although this study relates to the context of teaching online classes, their results do concur to the added value of student–educator relationships.

The following examples illustrate the relevance of teaching/learning caring relationships between nurse educators and their students in different situations:

- The teaching/learning caring relationship assists nurse educators to preserve students' human dignity, especially when learning challenges occur within the classroom.
- The teaching/learning caring relationship can initiate nurse educators to celebrate graduate students' success following oral presentations.
- The teaching/learning caring relationship can also guide nurse educators to help students find meaning related to their future profession even when they are being discouraged and are ready to quit their programs.

TIME OUT FOR REFLECTION

We invite you to write your reflection in a journal in order to link the preceding theoretical segment with your personal *teaching/learning caring relationship* developed with your students.

Think about a time when you were in a situation where it felt that you were in a teaching/learning caring relationship with one of your students, and then ask yourself the following questions:

- What was your lived experience of being in a teaching/learning caring relationship?
- What was it about the relationship that made it caring?
- How were you teaching your students?

- What did you learn from your students?
- What were the impacts for your students' learning? And for your teaching practice?

PRAGMATIC SEGMENT
A NURSING DOCTORAL STUDENT'S LIVED EXPERIENCE: THE SIGNIFICANCE OF TEACHING/LEARNING CARING RELATIONSHIPS

Houssem Eddine Ben Ahmed, PhD(c), MSc, RN, and Sylvain Brousseau, PhD, MSc, BSN, RN

This Pragmatic Segment describes a concrete example that elucidates the importance of establishing teaching/learning caring relationships in nursing education. The segment first illustrates a negative learning experience of an international doctoral student enrolled in a nursing program and then how teaching/learning caring relationships make a difference in the student's learning and academic success as well as the student's experience of his own teaching practice.

A Student's Lived Experience of Teaching/Learning Uncaring Relationships
In the student's first semester in the nursing doctoral program, as he started his first course in nursing science, he lived through a negative learning experience. He encountered an ongoing uncaring experience that made him feel anxious, stressed, and fearful, creating a lack of self-confidence and motivation to learn and to participate in group discussions in the classroom. There were various explanations of what could have caused this uncaring experience, such as social and cultural changes, different systems of education, favoritism toward certain students, and sarcastic comments during exams from some nurse educators, all dehumanizing practices in teaching/learning relationships that had physiological and psychological negative impacts on this student. Several studies have identified similar impacts (Arslan & Dinç, 2017;

Muliira, Natarajan, & van der Colff, 2017; Rawlins, 2017; Seibel & Fehr, 2018; Ziefle, 2018).

With respect to physiological impacts, the student developed a viral pathology that usually affects older people, caused by major stress and anguish during his first semester. Moreover, during the same semester, he gradually lost weight because of the uncaring relationships with some nurse educators. Unfortunately, such relationships are reported as still existing in our nursing schools. It has been acknowledged by Halldorsdottir (2013) as "life-restraining," one of the five basic modes of being with another. The negative experience also had psychological impacts on the student, such as having a feeling of anxiety and hopelessness during his first year in the program. Consequently, he became introverted and less involved in social life.

Fortunately, at that time, the student was well supported by his doctoral supervisors through his difficult academic process. Being informed by a humanistic caring perspective, such as described by Hills and Cara (2019) as well as Hills and Watson (2011), his doctoral supervisors gave all the support that he needed to succeed in his courses and his comprehensive exam, an important step in his doctoral program. These *teaching/learning caring relationships* between the student and his supervisors were characterized by a recognition of his uniqueness—as a unique human being and an international student. For example, in order to follow the student's learning progress more closely in his doctoral program, the supervisors recommended that they meet together at least three times per month to help with nursing science and philosophy. They also invited him to join them in some international conferences to learn to share his work with nursing scholars and to build his network. These relationships contributed not only to increasing the student's self-confidence but also to improving his scholarly progression.

In a teaching/learning situation, caring, or the lack of it, can have a significant impact on a student. Some nurse educators may consider caring as an inner behavior that does not need to be included into pedagogical practices and some do not encourage their students to invest much time to explore nursing education issues from a humanistic caring perspective. Still others, especially Paley (2002, p. 27), consider caring as a "slave morality" that prevents nursing from becoming a scientific discipline. From an opposing perspective, many scholars and students believe that caring is the essence of nursing education, which does not only concern the pedagogical content, such as teaching caring theories, but also focuses on developing teaching/learning relationships between students and educators. In agreement with Hills and Watson (2011) as well as Hills and Cara (2019), we consider that teaching/learning caring relationships between students and educators are a crucial component for the success of nursing education. For this reason, as Duffy (2018) pointed out, we highlight that caring relationships are a moral responsibility that educators should take into account in their pedagogical practices.

According to the present student's experience, establishing teaching/learning caring relationships with his supervisors contributed to his personal and professional development in the nursing doctoral program. The student felt more self-confident and more able to control his stress and anxiety during the first year of his nursing academic courses as a result of the caring relationships he was able to create with his supervisors. On the professional level, he became more committed in diverse activities such as attending national and international conferences, mentoring bachelor nursing students, and participating in scientific committees to evaluate scientific nursing abstracts. Indeed, all of this contributed to his empowerment and allowed him to develop networking with some experts and scholars in nursing, especially in nursing education.

It is also noteworthy that teaching/learning caring relationships are not only based on relational support between students and educators, but they also embrace rigorous pedagogical humanistic practices based on Caring Science. Educators should remain professional in their ways of teaching, acknowledging a student's personhood while being always guided by the humanistic caring perspective as recommended by Hills and Cara (2019). In this example, the student's doctoral supervisors were constantly rigorous during his different stages of writing his research proposal. Their caring attitudes and behaviors toward the doctoral student were expressed in various ways: by developing an authentic interaction, by formulating constructive comments, by encouraging him to undergo critical reflection, and sometimes by using humor. All these humanistic pedagogical strategies contributed to the advancement of his doctoral studies. Furthermore, as demonstrated in a qualitative study conducted by Froneman et al. (2016), these pedagogical practices, noted earlier, also strengthened the student's resilience in his doctoral program.

Student's Lived Experience of Teaching/Learning Caring Relationships in His Own Nursing Education Practice

Another recent concrete example that demonstrates the contribution of teaching/learning caring relationships to the success of nursing education is a student's own teaching experience as he was invited, along with another teaching assistant, to teach bachelor nursing students in a university. The doctoral student was very stressed because it was his first teaching experience. Before starting that, he asked the following questions:

- How should I start?
- Will students find my way of teaching interesting and enriching?
- Will my way of teaching contribute to their learning?
- How will I be able to foster nursing students' learning?

As a new teaching assistant, the doctoral student took some time to reflect about the best ways to teach students and to respond to those questions. Since he embraced a humanistic caring ontology as his pedagogical perspective, he decided to apply what he had learned and read about in Hills and Watson's (2011) Caring Science Curriculum in his process of teaching bachelor nursing students at the university. Before starting to teach, it was challenging for him to establish teaching/learning caring relationships with his students because, at that time, he recognized the importance to acknowledge the uniqueness of each student. In the process of teaching, the doctoral student found out that some bachelor students were very interested to learn new knowledge in nursing science, whereas others were not. He then perceived that his role, as a teaching assistant, was to nurture the motivated students and influence constructively the less-interested students.

First, the doctoral student asked his students to work in small groups in order to facilitate his interaction with them. Second, he asked them the following questions:

- How do they feel in the present moment?
- What does it mean to be in the present moment?

- Why are they here?
- What do they need to learn to become caring nurses?

These questions can lead undergraduate students to think ontologically about their "being a nursing student" and also motivate them to grasp the present moment the next time they meet in class. At the end of the first class, the doctoral student asked, "How did they find his way of teaching? How should he improve his teaching?" These questions and the students' comments helped the teaching assistant to learn and move to a further level of teaching. This method of establishing teaching/learning caring relationships distinguished him from the other teaching assistant who taught a different group of students. The teacher, responsible for the overall course, acknowledged that the doctoral student's group was very interested and concentrated in the classroom. In the other teacher assistant's group, some of the students were using their phones while others were sleeping or chatting on social media. We believe that nurse educators must manifest authenticity, loving presence, and openness, as well as recognize that involving students can make a difference in our transformational nursing educational world as described by Benner, Sutphen, Leonard, and Day (2010).

Teaching is a caring profession where educators have a critical and significant role in the lives of their students. We are reminded of Parker Palmer's (1997) words: "Good teaching cannot be reduced to technique; good teaching comes from the identity and integrity of the teacher" (p. 16). The circumstances recounted in this segment and in similar situations that seem all too prevalent are an urgent call to address dehumanizing practices as well as an invitation to nurse educators to reflect on teaching/learning caring relationships and reconsider their ways of teaching students.

CONCLUSION

This chapter intended to inform nurse educators on how to create and sustain *teaching/learning caring relationships* with students in order to improve students' learning of their future caring–healing practice as well as to cocreate knowledge. Those caring relationships are indeed fundamental to students learning their future praxis to promote patients' health, as they allow caring to be recognized, valued, and learned by students.

Moreover, the relational nature of nurse educators' work with students is crucial to humanize nursing education, as nurse educators' engagement and commitment in getting to know, understand, and accompany their students are required to develop these teaching/learning caring relationships. The nurse educators' moral imperative allows them to consider students, as unique individuals, at the center of their nursing programs. In other words, it is the teaching/learning caring relationships that contribute to transform teaching into a valuable human process.

REFERENCES

Arslan, S., & Dinç, L. (2017). Nursing students' perceptions of faculty members' ethical/unethical attitudes. *Nursing Ethics*, *24*(7), 789–801. doi:10.1177/0969733015625366

Beck, C. T. (2001). Caring within nursing education: A metasynthesis. *Journal of Nursing Education*, *40*(3), 101–109. doi:10.3928/0148-4834-20010301-04

Benner, P. (2005). Using the Dreyfus Model of Skill Acquisition to describe and interpret skill acquisition and clinical judgment in nursing practice and education. *The Bulletin of Science, Technology and Society*, *24*(3), 188–199. doi:10.1177/0270467604265061

Benner, P., Sutphen, M., Leonard, V., & Day, L. (2010). *Educating nurses: A call for radical transformation. The Carnegie report for the advancement of teaching*. San Francisco, CA: Jossey-Bass.

Bevis, E. O., & Watson, J. (1989). *Toward a caring curriculum: A new pedagogy for nursing*. New York, NY: National League for Nursing Press.

Bevis, E. O., & Watson, J. (2000). *Toward a caring curriculum: A new pedagogy for nursing* (2nd ed.). London, UK: Jones & Bartlett.

Boykin, A., Touhy, T. A., & Smith, M. C. (2011). Evolution of a caring-based college of nursing. In M. Hills & J. Watson. *Creating a Caring Science curriculum: An emancipatory pedagogy for nursing*. (pp. 157–184). New York, NY: Springer Publishing Company.

Cara, C., Gauvin-Lepage, J., Lefebvre, H., Létourneau, D., Alderson, M., Larue, C., … Mathieu, C. (2016). Le Modèle humaniste des soins infirmiers – UdeM: Perspective novatrice et pragmatique. *Recherche en soins infirmiers*, *125*, 20–31. doi:10.3917/rsi.125.0020

Cara, C., & Hills, M. (2018, May). *The added value of Caring Science: Its contributions to humanize nursing education*. Oral presentation at the Canadian Association of Schools in Nursing Conference, Montreal, QC, Canada.

Chan, Z. C., Tong, C. W., & Henderson, S. (2017). Power dynamics in the student-teacher relationship in clinical settings. *Nurse Education Today*, *49*, 174–179. doi:10.1016/j.nedt.2016.11.026

Duffy, J. (2018). *Quality caring in nursing and health professions, implications for clinicians, educators, and leaders* (3rd ed.). New York, NY: Springer Publishing Company.

Froneman, K., Du Plessis, E., & Koen, M. P. (2016). Effective educator-student relationships in nursing education to strengthen nursing students' resilience. *Curationis, 39*(1), 1595. doi:10.4102/curationis.v39i1.1595

Gillespie, M. (2005). Student–teacher connection: A place of possibility. *Journal of Advanced Nursing, 52*(2), 211–219. doi:10.1111/j.1365-2648.2005.03581.x

Grams, K., Kosowsky, M., & Wilson, C. (1997). Creating a caring community in nursing education. *Nurse Educator, 22*, 10–16. doi:10.1097/00006223-199705000-00011

Halldorsdottir, S. (1990). The essential structure of a caring and uncaring encounter with a teacher: The perspective of the nursing student. In M. Leininger & J. Watson (Eds.), *The caring imperative in nursing education* (pp. 95–108). New York, NY: National League for Nursing Press.

Halldorsdottir, S. (1991). Five basic modes of being with another. In D. A. Gaut & M. Leininger (Eds.), *Caring: The compassionate* (pp. 37–49). New York, NY: National League for Nursing Press.

Halldorsdottir, S. (2013). Five basic modes of being with another. In M. C. Smith, M. C. Turkel, & Z.R. Wolf (Eds.), *Caring in nursing classics: An essential resource* (pp. 201–210). New York, NY: Springer Publishing Company.

Hills, M., & Cara, C. (2019). Curriculum development processes and pedagogical practices for advancing Caring Science literacy. In W. Rosa, S. Horton-Deutsch, & J. Watson, (Eds.), *A handbook for Caring Science: Expanding the paradigm* (pp. 197–210). New York, NY: Springer Publishing Company.

Hills, M., & Watson, J. (2011). *Creating a Caring Science curriculum: An emancipatory pedagogy for nursing.* New York, NY: Springer Publishing Company.

Labrague, L. J., McEnroe-Petitte, D. M., Papathanasiou, I. V., Edet, O. B., & Arulappan, J. (2015). Impact of instructors' caring on students' perceptions of their own caring behaviors: Students' caring. *Journal of Nursing Scholarship, 47*(4), 338–346. doi:10.1111/jnu.12139

Miller, B. K., Haber, J., & Byrne, N. W. (1990). The experience of caring in the teaching process of nursing education: Student and teacher perspectives. In M. M. Leininger & J. Watson (Eds.), *The caring imperative in education* (pp. 255–266). New York, NY: National League for Nursing Press.

Muliira, J. K., Natarajan, J., & van der Colff, J. (2017). Nursing faculty academic incivility: Perceptions of nursing students and faculty. *BMC Medical Education, 17*(1), 1–10. doi:10.1186/s12909-017-1096-8

Noddings, N. (2012). The caring relation in teaching. *Oxford Review of Education, 38*(6), 771–781. doi:10.1080/03054985.2012.745047

Noddings, N. (2013). *Caring: A feminine approach to ethics and moral education* (2nd ed. updated). Berkeley: University of California Press.

Paley, J. (2002). Caring as a slave morality: Nietzschean themes in nursing ethics. *Journal of Advanced Nursing, 40*(1), 25–35. doi:10.1046/j.1365-2648.2002.02337.x

Palmer, J. P. (1997). The heart of a teacher identity and integrity in teaching. *Change: The Magazine of Higher Learning, 29*(6), 14–21. doi:10.1080/00091389709602343

Rawlins, L. (2017). Faculty and student incivility in undergraduate nursing education: An integrative review. *The Journal of Nursing Education, 56*(12), 709–716. doi:10.3928/01484834-20171120-02

Ray, M. A. (2010). *Transcultural caring dynamics in nursing and health care*. Philadelphia, PA: F. A. Davis.

Seibel, L. M., & Fehr, F. C. (2018). "They can crush you": Nursing students' experiences of bullying and the role of faculty. *Journal of Nursing Education and Practice, 8*(6), 66–76. doi:10.5430/jnep.v8n6p66

Sitzman, K., & Watson, J. (2017). *Watson's caring in the digital world: A guide for caring when interacting, teaching, and learning in cyberspace*. New York, NY: Springer Publishing Company.

Sitzman, K. L. (2007). Teaching-learning professional caring based on Jean Watson's theory of Human Caring. *International Journal of Human Caring, 11*(4), 8–16. doi:10.20467/1091-5710.11.4.8

Smith, Y. M., & Crowe, A. R. (2017). Nurse educator perceptions of the importance of relationship in online teaching and learning. *Journal of Professional Nursing, 33*(1), 11–19. doi:10.1016/j.profnurs.2016.06.004

Touhy, T., & Boykin, A. (2008). Caring as the central domain in nursing education. *International Journal for Human Caring, 12*(2), 8–15. doi:10.20467/1091-5710.12.2.8

Watson, J. (1999). *Postmodern nursing and beyond*. Edinburgh, UK: Churchill Livingstone.

Watson, J. (2000). A new paradigm of curriculum development. In E. O. Bevis & J. Watson (Eds.). *Toward a caring curriculum: A new pedagogy for nursing* (2nd ed., pp. 37–49). London, UK: Jones & Bartlett.

Watson, J. (2012). *Human Caring Science: A theory of nursing*. Sudbury, MA: Jones & Bartlett Learning.

Watson, J. (2018). *Unitary Caring Science. The philosophy and praxis of nursing*. Louisville: University of Colorado Press.

Whelan, J. (2017). The Caring Science imperative: A hallmark in nursing education. In S. Lee, P. Palmieri, & J. Watson (Eds.), *Global advances in Human Caring literacy* (pp. 33–42). New York, NY: Springer Publishing Company.

Ziefle, K. (2018). Incivility in nursing education: Generational differences. *Teaching and Learning in Nursing, 13*(1), 27–30. doi:10.1016/j.teln.2017.09.004

6

Caritas Processes and Caritas Literacy as a Teaching Guide for Enlightened Nurse Educators

As we enter into a maturing of Caring Science and evolved Caritas Processes *as a professional-theoretical map and guide, we are simultaneously challenged to relocate ourselves in these emerging ideals and ideas and question for ourselves how this work speaks to us as a discipline and a practice profession.*
—Watson, 2008, pp. 40–41

The named and researched human caring phenomena, ten Caritas Processes, have served as a philosophical-ethical theoretical guide to nursing caring-healing practices, both nationally and globally. These processes are considered universals of human caring, informed by the values and unitary worldview of Caring Science.
—Watson, 2018b, p. 54

LEARNING INTENTIONS

- Explore how nurse educators in their daily teaching/learning practices can be informed by Caritas Processes translated for nursing education.
- Recognize how the translated Teaching Caritas Processes can assist nurse educators to develop relationships with their students.

- Appreciate how the translated Teaching Caritas Processes and Caritas Literacy can contribute to humanize nursing education.
- Understand, from a nurse educator's and student's perspective, how the translated Teaching Caritas Processes can promote learning, development, and success for both persons involved.

INTRODUCTION

In this chapter, we explain how nurse educators can be informed by Caritas Processes and Caritas Literacy in their daily teaching/learning practices. These processes can serve nurse educators as a guide to develop caring relationships with their students, to assist and support their learning, which are fundamental in understanding how to become caring nurses. Before moving forward, we feel the need to define the term "literacy."

While the term usually corresponds with the capacity to read and write, in the context of Caring Science, it has a deeper meaning. Caring Science literacy "deepen[s] our ways of attending to and cultivating how to *Be-deeply Human/humane* and *Be-Caring* and Having a Healing presence. This form of *Being* is a form of human literacy, human artistry" (Watson, 2008, p. 23). This nursing theorist also explains that "being literate extends to the ability to incorporate concrete experience, experiential learning, context, and situations into one's life field. Thus, the term *literacy* has evolved to reflect the fact that there are multiple literacies" (Watson, 2017, p. 5). Therefore, Caritas Literacy embraces Watson's Caritas Processes as the nurse educators' guide to teach from a Caring Science perspective that can contribute to humanize nursing education.

WATSON'S CLINICAL CARITAS PROCESSES

Before discussing Watson's Caritas Processes, it seems necessary to explain what this theorist means by the term "Caritas."

> The term *Caritas* is from Latin, referring to that which is precious and cannot be taken for granted; it conveys charity in the sense of use of self in compassionate service to humankind. . . . Caritas [is used] to depict the deeper ethical philosophical value foundation of authentic professional human caring practice. . . . *Caritas* encompasses loving consciousness as the core of human caring—deepening the meaning of professional nurse [educator] caring beyond the outer slogan and trite use of the term *caring* . . . as a commodity to be bought and sold. (Watson, 2018b, pp. 73–74)

The significance and benefits of using Watson's Caritas Processes within clinical nursing practice have been mentioned by several authors (Cara, 2003; Cara & O'Reilly, 2008; Caruso, Cisar, & Pipe, 2008; Delmas, O'Reilly, Iglesias, Cara, & Burnier, 2016; Falk Rafael, 2000; O'Reilly, Cara, & Delmas, 2016; Perry & Cara, 2017; Sitzman, 2016; Sitzman & Watson, 2014). However, Watson's (2008, 2012, 2018b) Caritas Processes are not just noteworthy to nurses' or students' clinical practice. They can also guide nurse educators' strategies in their teaching/learning practices as well as in their interactions with their students. Indeed, they can enlighten nurse educators to assist and support their students' learning to become caring professionals. Therefore, this chapter aims to inform nurse educators on how to translate Watson's *Clinical Caritas Processes* into living *Teaching Caritas Processes*, informing nurse educators' teaching moral ideal related to their praxis with their students. Such praxis contributes to humanize nursing education.

TRANSLATED TEACHING CARITAS PROCESSES

Watson's (n.d.) Clinical Caritas Processes along with the translated processes for nurse educators, entitled "Teaching Caritas Processes," are shown in Table 6.1. Despite their interrelatedness, each Teaching Caritas Process will be presented distinctly in order to help nurse educators grasp how to apply each of them in their everyday teaching/learning practices.

However, before beginning, it is worth mentioning that Watson's work is grounded in a humanist philosophy. Such philosophy is thoroughly centered on the human being, in our instance, the students. According to Watson (2018b), humanistic values (e.g., those described in Chapter 2, Educators' Caring Values, Attitudes, and Behaviors That Contribute to the Humanization of Nursing Education) are essential to nurses' moral imperative in order to preserve humanity and Human Caring. With this perspective in mind, nurse educators will perceive each student with respect and consideration, as a complete person, hence a unique, whole, and holistic human being.

In other words, the Teaching Caritas Processes point to a different way of knowing, doing, being, and becoming a caring nurse educator to accompany students in learning their future caring practice for patients, families, and communities—that is, learning to teach from the heart, with passion and love for students and nursing (see also Chapter 4, Humanizing Nursing Education by Teaching From the Heart).

Table 6.1 Watson's Caritas Processes Translated for Nurse Educators

Clinical Caritas Processes	Translated Teaching Caritas Processes
1) Sustaining humanistic–altruistic values by practice of loving-kindness, compassion, and equanimity with self/others	1) Sustaining humanistic–altruistic values by the practice of loving-kindness, compassion, and equanimity **in teaching/learning practices** with self **and students**
2) Being authentically present, enabling faith/hope/belief system; honoring subjective inner, life-world of self/others	2) Being authentically present **in teaching/learning practices**, enabling faith/hope/belief system; honoring subjective inner, life-world of self **and students**
3) Being sensitive to self and others by cultivating own spiritual practices; beyond ego-self to transpersonal presence	3) Being sensitive to self and **students** by cultivating own spiritual practices; beyond ego-self to transpersonal presence **in teaching/learning practices**
4) Developing and sustaining loving, trusting-caring relationships	4) Developing and sustaining loving, trusting-caring relationships **with students**
5) Allowing for expression of positive and negative feelings—authentically listening to another person's story	5) Allowing for expression of positive and negative feelings—authentically listening to **the student's** story
6) Creatively problem-solving-"solution-seeking" through caring process; full use of self and artistry of caring–healing practices via use of all ways of knowing/being/doing/becoming	6) Creatively problem-solving-"solution-seeking" through caring process; full use of self and artistry of caring–healing **teaching/learning** practices via use of all ways of knowing/being/doing/becoming
7) Engaging in transpersonal teaching and learning within context of caring relationship; staying within other's frame of reference-shift toward coaching model for expanded health/wellness	7) Engaging in transpersonal teaching and learning within context of caring **educator–student** relationship; staying within **the student's** frame of reference-shift toward coaching model for expanded **learning/meaning**

(continued)

Table 6.1 **Watson's Caritas Processes Translated for Nurse Educators** *(Continued)*

Clinical Caritas Processes	Translated Teaching Caritas Processes
8) Creating a healing environment at all levels; subtle environment for energetic authentic caring presence	8) Creating a healing **teaching/ learning** environment at all levels; subtle environment for energetic authentic caring **educator–student** presence
9) Reverentially assisting with basic needs as sacred acts, touching mindbodyspirit of spirit of other; sustaining human dignity	9) Reverentially assisting with basic **students' cognitive and spiritual learning** needs as sacred acts, touching mindbodyspirit of spirit of other; sustaining **students'** human dignity
10) Opening to spiritual, mystery, unknowns—allowing for miracles	10) Opening to spiritual, mystery, unknowns—allowing for miracles **to enter teaching/learning practices**

Source: Watson, J. (n.d.). *10 Caritas Processes®*. Watson Caring Science Institute. Retrieved from https://www .watsoncaringscience.org/jean-bio/caring-science-theory/10-caritas-processes

First Teaching Caritas Process

The first Teaching Caritas Process, *Sustaining humanistic–altruistic values by the practice of loving-kindness, compassion, and equanimity in teaching/ learning practices with self and students*, is twofold. Despite the fact that both portions are intertwined, we discuss each separately.

The first part concerns the nurse educator's *humanistic–altruistic values*. Besides referring to Chapter 2, Educators' Caring Values, Attitudes, and Behaviors That Contribute to the Humanization of Nursing Education, pertaining to humanistic values (e.g., respect, human dignity, and believing in the students' potential), the humanistic–altruistic values are, according to Watson (2008), grounded in kindness, gentleness, compassion, concern, and love for, in our case, our students and colleagues, our teaching/learning practices, our social mission, our discipline and profession, as well as humanity. Hence, it implies a profound desire to help and assist students in their learning of the discipline and profession. For example, this first Teaching Caritas Process may guide nurse educators to be concerned and available to accompany students presenting some difficulties to understand the class assignment or to take the time to assist international graduate students to better grasp the academic culture of the graduate nursing program.

In addition, embracing humanistic–altruistic values, according to Sitzman and Watson (2014, p. 43), is also associated with a "nonharming [sic] and having a desire to help" attitude. This means that in the case of nursing education, nurse educators are adopting a humanistic attitude and are genuinely concerned about students' learning, well-being, and safety. Concretely, to adopt a humanistic attitude can also be revealed by nurse educators being considerate in the way they formulate their evaluation and critique of students' realizations. In other words, nurse educators will use "constructive" criticisms rather than "destructive" criticisms. This also means to focus on students' strengths rather than just concentrating on their weaknesses. For example, when grading a paper, caring nurse educators will write positive feedback to motivate and support students' efforts. Truly, teachers can discourage students with harsh, negative, and devastating comments. As Noddings (2013) mentions, "punitive moves work against the development of subjective responsibility that is required for continuous construction of the ethical ideal. They give the wrong message about both intellectual work and our relations to each other" (p. 201). Indeed, nurse educators are instrumental in students' learning as they can nurture them or destroy them while providing feedback. Bevis (2000a) suggests rather nurturing students, their caring role, their creativity, their curiosity, as well as their assertiveness within their learning journey. Such nurturance from nurse educators corresponds to exhibiting these humanistic–altruistic values, substantially contributing to humanize nursing education.

The second part of this first Teaching Caritas Process, *practice of loving-kindness, compassion, and equanimity in teaching/learning practices with self and students*, starts with oneself. Indeed Watson (2008) explicates that "[c]aring begins with being present, open to compassion, mercy, gentleness, loving-kindness, and equanimity toward and with self before one can offer compassionate caring to others" (p. xviii). Consequently, Watson (2008) explains that equanimity is required to reach such Caritas consciousness in order to be caring with others. She defines equanimity as a sense of inner balance, allowing oneself to be in harmony. Indeed, this first process invites "nurses to attend to self-caring and practices that assist in their own evolution of consciousness for more fulfillment in their life and work. In this way of thinking, nurses [educators] can be models and living exemplars" (Watson,

2008, p. 47). Nurse educators' self-caring activities are seldom considered in nursing schools, unless teaching within a Caring Science Curriculum (Hills & Watson, 2011).

Additionally, nurse educators' loving-kindness attitudes toward students could entail diverse expressions and behaviors grounded in a deep aspiration to love, care, and help out in any meaningful ways (Watson, 2018a; see also Chapter 4, Humanizing Nursing Education by Teaching From the Heart). For example, in nursing education, Rockwood Lane and Samuels (2011) suggest nurse educators symbolize their classroom as a caring community, where each student is cared for and honored with acceptance, tolerance, and humanness. Hence, being informed by this Teaching Caritas Process, nurse educators can request students to be kind to their colleagues and to provide feedback in a helpful way in order to be supportive and encouraging. Creating a caring climate in their classroom (which is also related to the eighth Teaching Caritas Process) will also help students to learn how to be supportive rather than competitive with one another. This experiential learning can be useful in their future practice in order to be supportive of healthcare professionals and staff. Indeed, several authors have mentioned that students can learn tremendously about caring through their caring interaction with their peers (Beck, 2001; Hughes, 1993) as well as with their teachers (Beck, 2001; Cara, 2001; Cara et al., 2016; Chan, Tong, & Henderson, 2017; Cook & Cullen, 2003; Froneman, Du Plessis, & Koen, 2016; Gillespie, 2005; Halldorsdottir, 1990; Hills & Watson, 2011; Labrague, McEnroe-Petitte, Papathanasiou, Edet, & Arulappan, 2015; Murray, 2000; Noddings, 2012, 2013; Whelan, 2017; Wiklund-Gustin & Wagner, 2013).

According to Watson (2008), to practice from this first Caritas Process can be developed only through a profound self-consciousness (see also Chapter 3, Emancipatory Contributions to Humanize Nursing Education). In other words, through a close examination of one's own beliefs and one's own values, nurse educators can aspire to personal and professional growth, fulfillment, and transformation. Subsequently, such teaching/learning Caritas practice can transform both nurse educators and students. Indeed, both can grasp, understand, experience, and foster their awareness concerning their caring role and their caring praxis.

This first Teaching Caritas Process can also serve to guide nurse educators to expand their worldview and consciousness regarding the relational nature of their role. Certainly, being inspired by Human Caring can expand nurse educators' consciousness on how to relate to students, in order to guide them and share their learning venture. Ultimately, caring as a moral ideal can assist nurse educators to become the best teachers possible in order to potentiate students' learning and development. As Watson (2012) reports,

> a moral ideal for nursing [education allows nurse educators] to call on the inner depth of their own humanness and personal creativity as they realize the conditions of a [student's] soul and their own. . . . The transpersonal human-to-human caring is the essence and moral ideal of a style of nursing [education] where human dignity and humanity are preserved and human indignity is alleviated in health-illness [teaching/learning] experiences. (p. 85)

Second Teaching Caritas Process

The second Teaching Caritas Process, *Being authentically present in teaching/learning practices, enabling faith/hope/belief system; honoring subjective inner, life-world of self and students*, is threefold. Despite the fact that all three parts are linked together, we explain each individually for more clarity. The first part of this Teaching Caritas Process, *being authentically present in teaching/learning practices*, pertains to nurse educators' authentic presence within their teaching/learning practices, in order to instill faith-hope and honor their students. According to Watson (2018b), an "authentic presence" between two persons, in our case the nurse educator and the student, captures a special type of connection: a human-to-human, a heart-to-heart, and a spirit-to-spirit encounter. By perceiving nurse educators' authentic presence, students will be more likely to feel their teachers' concern for their learning and development. Although it is possible to experience and recognize such an encounter, it is also possible to perceive its absence. Also, such an authentic presence is closely connected with openness, caring consciousness, and mindfulness, as explained by Watson (2008):

> By being sensitive to our own [teaching] presence and *Caritas Consciousness*, not only are we able to offer and enable another to access his or her own belief system of faith-hope for the person's healing [students' learning], but we may be the one who makes the difference between hope and despair in a given [teaching] moment. (p. 62)

The second part of this Teaching Caritas Process, *enabling faith/hope/belief system*, may guide nurse educators to instigate a positive attitude among the students toward their own success within the nursing program. For example, nurse educators guided by this Teaching Caritas Process will inspire their students to have faith in themselves, their intellectual abilities, their cognitive capacities, their reasoning aptitudes, their critical thinking, as well as their procedural skills. The nurse educators will also focus on students' assets, not only their weaknesses or inadequacy, in order to facilitate established goals that the class agreed upon at the beginning of the semester. Watson (2008) reminds nurses of the healing power of faith, hope, and belief for a person. In other words, it is hope that can carry a student to succeed when failure is likely to happen. Said differently, this Teaching Caritas Process may guide nurse educators in being present to their students and making a difference in their learning journey by instilling faith and hope that they can reach an academic success in the nursing program.

The third part of this Teaching Caritas Process, *honoring subjective inner, life-world of self and students*, implies that nurse educators will honor their students' deep beliefs and meanings throughout their learning endeavor. As explained by Watson (2008),

> [i]n *Caritas Consciousness*, the nurse [educator] honors and seeks to dis-cover what is meaningful and important for a particular [student]. The [student's] beliefs are never discarded or dismissed as insignificant in the [nurse educator's caring teaching/learning practices]. Indeed, they are encouraged, respected, and enabled as significant in promoting [learning and development] and wholeness. (p. 65)

Hence, being informed by this second Teaching Caritas Process, nurse educators are invited to ask their students to share their beliefs, meanings, fears, and questions regarding their future caring practices. Nurse educators may also instill faith in regard to students' future caring practice by sharing stories on how caring is beneficial for patients, families, and communities as well as for nurses themselves. In fact, Bevis and Watson (1989, 2000) believe that narrative strategies are relevant in order to raise students' consciousness concerning nursing societal mandate (see also Chapter 3, Emancipatory Contributions to Humanize Nursing Education).

Related to this Caritas Process, Sitzman and Watson (2014) mention that "being authentically present, instilling faith and hope, and honoring others require caring [nurse educators] to cultivate openness to, and awareness of, alternative practices and beliefs" (p. 55). With that in mind, and adapted to nursing education, the authors suggest nurse educators be open to alterna-tive pedagogical strategies and ideas, which will be further explained with the seventh Teaching Caritas Process.

As mentioned earlier, this second Teaching Caritas Process is also valu-able when students are experiencing a failing situation. For example, nurse educators, guided by this Teaching Caritas Process, will encourage students to keep hope; we are referring here not to a false self-confidence but to a realistic hope. In such a case, nurse educators would assist students in finding goals to improve academically. Concretely, it would be suggested that both students along with nurse educators plan tangible and realistic goals in order to meet each of the evaluation criteria. However, it is essential to address students' difficulties as soon as possible in the semester, as it is much more difficult for students to improve the situation at the very end of the semester when almost nothing can any longer be done.

Third Teaching Caritas Process

The third Teaching Caritas Process, *Being sensitive to self and students by cultivating own spiritual practices; beyond ego-self to transpersonal presence in teaching/learning practices*, guides nurse educators not only to be self-aware but also to assist students in acknowledging their personal and professional beliefs, emotions, and reactions within every step of their learning journey.

According to Sitzman and Watson (2014), this specific "Caritas Process makes clear that professionally mature caring–healing comportment is dependent upon personal cultivation of deep knowing and doing" (p. 65). In other words, this Teaching Caritas Process is fundamental to uphold students' caring practice by encouraging both introspection and reflective practice to take place. In their work, Rockwood Lane and Samuels (2011) propose to "create rituals that allow students to become connected to their own experience and what they bring to the class" (p. 221). They also give ideas on how to create such rituals in the class. For example, they propose guided imagery, meditation, or writing letters or poetry to facilitate their students' introspection.

Consequently, nurse educators being guided by this third Teaching Caritas Process will not consider students as simply reduced to the moral status of an "object," to be filled up with information, but rather consider them as whole and unique human beings, in relation with the world (both personally and professionally). In fact, to distinguish students' personal spheres is relevant since it can be advantageous for nurse educators to be aware of students' personal beliefs and experiences about both natural and professional caring practice in order to accompany them in a reflective practice (either individually or collectively).

Also, linked to this third Teaching Caritas Process is the acknowledgment of students' spiritual dimension and internal power of the teaching/learning caring process, growth, and transformation. It is often challenging to address "spirituality" in clinical settings, yet again in nursing education. To appreciate students' spiritual dimension is to acknowledge their "spiritual–inner subjective life world" (Watson, 2012, p. 88). Concretely, nurse educators may accompany their students to understand their spirituality, or they may even explore their own spirituality. For example, by performing reflective practice or journaling, they can identify their own existential beliefs, their quest for meaning in their personal and professional lives, their connectedness with self and others as well as their inner force and motivation within their learning journey. Hence, it is also to concede that students have personal beliefs and values that will be part of their learning of the nursing discipline and profession.

Lastly, inspired by this Teaching Caritas Process, nurse educators will also promote and nurture their own actualization by appreciating their own feelings and fostering their personal growth as caring teachers. As Watson (2008) explains this Caritas Process remains a lifelong evolving adventure of learning to be able to teach, in this case, to our students. She clarifies that

> without attending to and cultivating one's own spiritual growth, insight, mindfulness, and spiritual dimension of life, it is very difficult to be sensitive to self and other. Without this lifelong process and journey, we can become hardened and brittle and can close down our compassion and caring for self and other. Thus, this *Caritas Process* seeks to make explicit that our professional commitment to caring-healing and the wholeness of Being/doing/knowing cannot be complete or mature without focusing on this evolving aspect of our personal and professional growth. (pp. 67–68)

In fact, Benner, Sutphen, Leonard, and Day (2010) as well as Hills and Watson (2011) also encourage teachers' reflective practice. For example, Benner et al. (2010) argued that nurse educators rarely have the opportunity to reflect on their own teaching practice as well as its improvement or transformation. These authors suggest supporting opportunities to "learn and demonstrate exemplary teaching" in order to promote students' learning (p. 224). Thus, an individual and collective reflective practice is essential to describe, understand, analyze, critique, and enrich one's caring praxis (Cara, 2014; Cara et al., 2016). For example, inspired by Payette and Champagne's work (1997) on "professional codevelopment group approach," nurse educators can be invited to gather in order to discuss how to improve their own professional teaching practice. This group would share a culture of learning and caring, so as to listen, support, and discover from each other, cherishing each other's perspectives, experiences, skills, strengths, and expertise.

As Payette and Champagne (1997) explain, the commitment to the professional codevelopment group provides important incentive, motivation, and cohesion to share, reflect, express, and learn from each other and together. Such a professional codevelopment group approach should bring empowerment and transformation to nurse educators' teaching/learning practices.

Fourth Teaching Caritas Process

The fourth Teaching Caritas Process, *Developing and sustaining loving, trusting-caring relationships with students*, corresponds to the very heart of the educator–student learning/teaching relationship (see also Chapter 5, Seeking Teaching/Learning Caring Relationships With Students). As previously mentioned, the relationships taking place between nurse educators and students are central to students' learning.

According to Watson (2008), it is the caring relationships that protect humanity, human dignity, and wholeness of human beings, in our case, students. Moreover, educator–student relationships would be considered "caring" because of nurse educators' Caritas consciousness, mindfulness, intentionality, loving-kindness, and presence to students.

> It conveys a concern for the inner life world and subjective meaning of [the student]; that other is fully embodied, that is, embodied spirit. . . . [The nurse educator] is more able to enter into and stay within the [student's] frame of reference; . . . to attend to what is most important for the [student] behind [the content and the teaching strategies]. The nurse [educator] is alert and responsive to what is present and emerging for the [student] in this given-now-moment. (Watson, 2008, p. 79)

Being inspired by Watson's (2008) work to reach an educator–students caring relationship, it is suggested that both, nurse educators and students, honor each other as unique human beings (see also Chapter 5, Seeking Teaching/Learning Caring Relationships With Students). It is also important to be able to verbalize and listen without any judgment, but rather with compassion. Additionally, both nurse educators and students can come to realize that they share each other's journey toward learning, development, transformation, and empowerment.

Furthermore, this Teaching Caritas Process guides nurse educators to demonstrate specific caring attitudes that provide an appropriate context to inspire students' learning and development. Here are some attitudes that the nurse educators can have: compassion, presence, openness, accessibility, active listening, authenticity, understanding, and so forth (also refer to Chapter 2, Educators' Caring Values, Attitudes, and Behaviors That Contribute to the Humanization of Nursing Education). As Cara, O'Reilly, and Brousseau (2017) explain, a caring ontology invites each person's subjectivity through advocacy, openness, commitment, compassion, and presence, henceforth enabling dialogue, mutuality, and relationship. Concretely, nurse educators' genuineness, consciousness, and concern for students and self are essential to enable trust within the teaching/ learning relationships, which is crucial to support learning and students' emancipation. In other words, caring nurse educators are committed to establish a trusting relationship with students. Such trust appears essential in nursing education so that students can feel safe to learn, ask questions, share their preoccupations, critique ideas, and cocreate knowledge through a respectful dialogue.

Fifth Teaching Caritas Process

The fifth Teaching Caritas Process, *Allowing for expression of positive and negative feelings—authentically listening to the student's story*, appears to be linked to the fourth Caritas Process. Indeed, to create an educator–student helping and trusting relationship, the nurse educator and the student need to be open and supportive of each other's expressions of positive and negative feelings. Inspired by this Teaching Caritas Process, nurse educators need to offer a caring and safe environment in order to encourage students to express, particularly, their negative feelings. Usually, positive feelings are very well received by people. However, negative feelings are not so easy to invite, allow, endorse, and support. So, being inspired by this Teaching Caritas Process can guide nurse educators to be nonjudgmental and receptive while listening to their students' negative feelings. As Watson (2008) states, there is no right or wrong feelings, but just feelings to receive, acknowledge, and honor. She believes that such a caring and open attitude will help create mutual trust and understanding within the relationship. In fact, students' feedback is significant for educators' reflective teaching/learning practices (also see Chapter 3, Emancipatory Contributions to Humanize Nursing Education, and Chapter 7, Habitus: An Ontological Space Fostering Humanistic Nursing Education).

For example, students must feel safe to express their interrogations, their anxiety, their feelings, their understanding, their difficulties, their struggles, their distress, along with their vulnerability. Indeed, during class, content related, for example to death and palliative care, may bring up emotional reactions, anxiety, discomfort, or even suffering. Hence, students would most likely benefit from being accompanied by nurse educators to find meaning in their vulnerability and suffering. Confidentiality must also be respected in order for students to feel safe to share and learn within the classroom. According to Rockwood Lane and Samuels (2011), students are asked to "create a commitment that honors every student's story. The sharing is confined to the classroom, which allows students to know they are safe in their vulnerabilities if and when they choose to share" (p. 222).

Besides, for students, expressing their feelings will also help them to become self-aware and reflective about their own nursing practice. In order to promote this, nurse educators can invite, for example, their students to write a journal or a story where they can reflect on their caring practice as well as their learning and progress. Such an exercise can assist students to seek a deeper understanding of the knowledge to be learned. According to Benner et al. (2010), journaling promotes students' (and nurse educators' for that matter) discovery, learning, and knowledge integration, as well as sharing of their experiential clinical learning. In other words, such activities will contribute to their reflective practice and to seek personal meaning. Additionally, Hills and Watson (2011) suggest that journaling and writing narratives, as exemplars from their practices, will help develop a culture of caring within the classroom.

Sixth Teaching Caritas Process

The sixth Teaching Caritas Process, *Creatively problem-solving-"solution-seeking" through caring process; full use of self and artistry of caring-healing teaching/learning practices via use of all ways of knowing/being/doing/becoming*, can guide nurse educators in their daily teaching. It invites nurse educators to ground their students' support and learning/teaching practices not only on a scientific approach to problem-solving but on all ways of knowing (Carper, 1978; Chinn & Kramer, 2018), on creativity, as well as Human Caring.

More specifically, drawing from Carper's (1978) initial work, Chinn and Kramer (2018) identify the following ways of knowing as being essential to our nursing discipline: emancipatory, ethics, empirics, personal, as well as aesthetic. While using all ways of knowing, Watson (2008) clarifies that nurse [educators] have to gain insight, experience, and understanding in order to proceed with their decision-making.

Moreover, Watson (2008) explains that

> [t]he complexity of decision making and acting within *Caritas Processes* requires critical thinking, clarity of rationale, and use of scientific

evidence; but it also demands a focus and an orientation that make explicit the multifaceted creative, integrative, critical thinking necessary for engaging in a systematic, synthesized problem-solving focus for an individualized [student's learning] situation. (p. 114)

Hence, Watson (2008) argues that this Caritas Process is neither systematic nor linear. She states that "[t]he evolved *Caritas Nurse* [educator] celebrates the caring process as a creative, intuitive, aesthetic, ethical, personal, even spiritual process, as well as a professional empirical-technical process" (p. 107).

Therefore, guided by this Teaching Caritas Process, nurse educators are invited to truly comprehend the situation, using all ways of knowing, to decide the best pedagogical interventions, understanding not only the class objectives and the projected competencies but also their students' lived experience. Nurse educators are invited to know self and others as a caring person in order to comprehend and explore new solutions to difficulties from a Human Caring perspective. Hence, the use of self is particularly important in this sixth Caritas Process (Watson, 2008).

In other words, this Teaching Caritas Process assists nurse educators to identify students' needs and preoccupations, plan their pedagogical activities in partnership with the students when possible, teach interactively, reevaluate the situation, as well as invite students' feedback to inform their reflective teaching practice.

Seventh Teaching Caritas Process

The seventh Teaching Caritas Process corresponds to *Engaging in transpersonal teaching and learning within context of caring educator–student relationship; staying within the student's frame of reference-shift toward coaching model for expanded learning/meaning*. This particular Caritas Process stands especially relevant to nurse educators in their pedagogical interventions as well as their learning/teaching praxis. This Teaching Caritas Process is twofold. Despite the fact that both segments are interlaced, we discuss each separately.

As previously declared, we believe that it is no longer enough to teach the content to students as they are passively learning. According to Watson (2008), and as stated earlier, teaching involves a genuine and caring relationship based on trust, which respects the individual as a whole person (see the fourth Teaching Caritas Process as well as Chapter 5, Seeking Teaching/Learning Caring Relationships With Students). Therefore, from nurse educators' experience, authenticity, meaning, and relationship, their teaching process will become genuine as well as transpersonal, ultimately influencing both oneself and the student. Beck (2001) recognizes the following uplifting effects of caring in education: "being respected, belonging, growth, transformed, learning to care, and a desire to care. Experiencing caring from a faculty member or nursing student results in feeling valued and respected as a unique person" (p. 107).

Moreover, we believe that the educator–student caring relationship must be informed by consciousness, intentionality, as well as open communication (see also Chapter 3, Emancipatory Contributions to Humanize Nursing Education). Indeed, intentionality is essential for nurse educators in order to focus on assisting students to learn about the nursing discipline and profession. As Watson (1999) explains, "the transformative consciousness, intentionality and energy connection, as part of a broader ethic and choice among health professions, offers new considerations and new awakenings to the nature of our being in a relationship with one who is in need" (p. 128). In other words, nurse educators must be consciously aware that they wish to develop a caring relationship with their students in order to assist them in their learning and development. Besides, educators' awareness and consciousness originate from their teaching moral ideal, wanting to be the best teacher possible. Indeed, nurse educators' moral ideal upholds their concern for students' human dignity as well as the preservation of humanity in general. Associated with nursing education, one can understand the preservation of humanity as being part of the teachers' social mandate (Bevis & Watson, 1989, 2000; Brown, 2011; Cook & Cullen, 2003; Hills & Watson, 2011).

Additionally, this Caritas Process invites nurse educators' commitment to genuine teaching/learning experiences within relationships with their students, while acknowledging the necessity of staying within their frame of reference. To be in the other's frame of reference is crucial, according to Watson (2008), in order to move on to the level of Caritas Coach. In sync with this Teaching Caritas Process, nurse educators will consider the students' perspectives, past lived experiences, perceptions, and meanings in order to address their learning needs. Concretely, nurse educators are invited to be perceptive and sensitive to students' perspectives so to assist them in finding meaning in the new knowledge learned. Without this approach, some students might be less likely to be motivated to receive, process, and analyze the information to grasp meanings relevant to caring for patients, families, and communities.

With that in mind, nurse educators are encouraged to be open to alternative pedagogical strategies and ideas. Several authors also advocate nontraditional, integrative or emancipatory teaching, and learning pedagogical approaches (Benner et al., 2010; Bevis & Watson, 1989, 2000; Boykin, Touhy, & Smith, 2011; Chinn & Kramer, 2018; Goudreau et al., 2009; Hills & Watson, 2011; Labrague et al., 2015; Touhy & Boykin, 2008). Indeed, a traditional lecture format, oriented mostly on facts, principles, diseases, and interventions, is not optimal for students to acquire knowledge. Rather, students' learning is most likely to occur within a caring atmosphere, which promotes dialogue, debate, and reflection in regard to the study of various nursing situations lived by patients, families, and communities. Likewise, in their correlational study pertaining to the impact of instructors' caring behaviors on students' perceptions related to their own caring behaviors, Labrague et al. (2015) conclude that

> nursing curricula should incorporate teaching strategies grounded in the ethic of caring, which promotes caring values in student nurses. Students' engagement in learning caring may be fostered through nontraditional learning pedagogy such as simulations, educational games, and the use of patients' narratives in order to bring reality to classroom settings where caring could be explored. (p. 7)

These authors also suggest role-playing as an effective teaching strategy for students to understand experientially what caring really means for them.

Certainly, nurse educators are requested to ask themselves the following question: Teaching for what end in view? (Bevis, 2000a, p. 154). Considering the education's social mandate, giving passively the content, or as Bevis (2000a) explains, absorption, memorization, and recitation of the information, is simply not enough. Indeed, nurse educators are invited to challenge students to raise meaningful questions pertaining to their patients' lived experiences, inquire with all ways of knowing to better understand their situation, and engage in critical thinking in order to decide, along with their patients, the best interventions that will promote health and healing, as well as respect their human dignity.

Bevis (2000b) also reveals the following "scholarly modalities" pertaining to the students' learning process aimed to "enable" their learning:

- "Analysis"
- "Critiquing"
- "Recognizing insights"
- "Identifying and evaluating assumptions"
- "Inquiring into the nature of things"
- "Projecting, futuring, anticipating, predicting, or hypothesizing"
- "Engaging in praxis"

- "Viewing wholes, not just parts in relation to each other"
- "Finding meanings in ideas and experiences" (pp. 235–236)

Furthermore, Bevis (2000b) also suggests nurse educators assist their students in developing learning tools, which she calls "educational heuristics," so as to guide their learning experience (p. 236). This concept of "heuristics" means to enable students to discover something for themselves and to learn from finding their personal meaning. For example, she proposes the following "educational heuristics" (Bevis, 2000b):

- "Reflection"
- "Discussion, dialogue, and debate"
- "[I]maging, imagining, and envisioning"
- "Intuiting, hunching"
- "Tracing logical pathways" (p. 237)

We believe this approach to be the opposite of the traditional behavioral model, where students are most likely rewarded for their acquiescence, conformity, and adherence to the nurse educators' point of view. Concretely, using this heuristic approach, nurse educators wanting to teach about breast cancer could ask students to start their learning process from their own personal or professional experience before reading textbooks or scientific papers in order to better integrate women's lived experience of suffering from breast cancer.

Additionally, Hills and Watson (2011) also consider "critical dialogue," an underpinning of their emancipatory relational pedagogy, as crucial to promote students' learning:

> Critical dialogue consists of three essential interwoven processes and elements: listening, critical questioning, and critical thinking. . . . The main purpose of critical dialogue is to create opportunities for critical thinking and critical reflection that result in the creation of new understandings (knowledge). Always transformative, critical dialogue aims to put teachers and students in situations where they *encounter* preconceived notions and ideas in ways that encourage them to question their assumptions. Without this type of encounter, they may be engaged in a discussion, but it would not be a critical caring dialogue. (pp. 87–88)

Also, this Teaching Caritas Process incites nurse educators to be in sync with students' rhythm or pace of learning. Nurse educators have to remember that each student's learning experience is unique. As explained by Watson (2008), it is important to pay attention to the learners' context, needs, interests, learning styles, as well as their readiness to learn. In fact, being in sync with the students' rhythm can make a difference in their acquiring as well as their understanding of new knowledge.

Lastly, we perceive students as coparticipants within the teaching/learning caring process. The term "coparticipant" is significant for both the student and the educator. Coparticipation requires cooperation and dialogue in order to keep the communication open between nurse educators and students. Therefore, coparticipation appears to be tremendously important, otherwise no partnership or relationship can occur. "Participation requires commitment. It is a conscious decision to devote time, energy, and resources to teaching/learning. Participation demands engagement" (Hills & Watson, 2011, p. 80). As for the coparticipants' engagement, it is illustrated by their concern, openness, and presence. In other words, Beck (2001) explains that

> authentic presencing sets the stage for caring to unfold in nursing education. Presencing one's self centers on striving to enter the world of the other—the world of a faculty member, nursing student, or patient. Attentive listening is crucial to achieving presencing. . . . When "tuned in" to the other person, words are not needed to convey the need for caring. . . . Authentic presencing is the start of a personal, intimate process of caring. (p. 104)

Hence, such nurse educators' presence is fundamental to work within the students' frame of reference, which is required to being and becoming a Caritas Coach for students throughout their learning journey.

Eighth Teaching Caritas Process

The eighth Teaching Caritas Process, *Creating a healing teaching/learning environment at all levels; subtle environment for energetic authentic caring educator–student presence*, discusses how students are interdependent with the teaching/learning environment. Inspired by this Teaching Caritas Process in the nursing education realm, nurse educators will promote, through their support, students' harmony of being-in-the-world as part of their nursing program.

Hills and Watson (2011) as well as Touhy and Boykin (2008) explicate that a caring atmosphere promotes an open dialogue, discussion, argumentation, and different ways of knowing for both nurse educators and students. Indeed, according to Touhy and Boykin (2008), "teaching and learning occur through open dialogue and reflection rather than in a lecture format where facts and principles are presented" (p. 9). In her metasynthesis on caring within nursing education, Beck (2001) concludes that the creation of a caring environment is critical not only for teaching students how to care for patients but also to develop relationships and cohesion among both students and nursing teachers.

Guided by this Teaching Caritas Process, nurse educators will encourage students' comfort and safety within the learning environment, taking into account their strengths and weaknesses related to learning. For example, Rockwood Lane and Samuels (2011) suggest creating a classroom environment that is noncritical and nonjudgmental, "a sacred space," so as to embrace students' creativity and experimentation. In so doing, nurse educators will support the students' learning experiences and encourage them to be caring and supportive of each other. Such an environment can be considered "healing" when it symbolizes wholeness, elegance, comfort, privacy, and beauty (Watson, 1999).

In addition, Watson (2008) explains that "holding authentic, heartfelt, positive thoughts such as loving-kindness, caring, healing, forgiveness, and so forth, vibrates at a higher level [of energy] than having lower thoughts, such as competition, fear, greed, anxiety, hostility . . . The [nurse educator] . . . *Becomes* the environment, affecting the entire field" (p. 140).

Lastly, nurse educators are encouraged to expand their mode of consciousness beyond the traditional behaviorist paradigm, toward a postmodern paradigm, which is linked with Human Caring. Several authors also acknowledge the need for a paradigm shift in nursing education (Bevis & Watson, 1989, 2000; Brown, 2011; Cara & Hills, 2018; Cara, Hills, & Watson, 2019; Hills & Cara, 2019; Hills & Watson, 2011; National League for Nursing, 2003).

> Within the postmodern/transpersonal framework, nursing arts, skills, or "fundamentals" remain "essential," but for entirely different reasons. For once one has an expanded consciousness and a different intentionality, it is no longer appropriate, nor acceptable, to engage in technical, routine, body-physical care, administered as a job "to get done," as people who need "to be done," as techniques to be mechanically and technically completed to persons as bodies. Something new has to transpire in the practitioner. (Watson, 1999, p. 240)

Watson's quote might be particularly relevant while teaching technical skills to students.

Ninth Teaching Caritas Process

The ninth Teaching Caritas Process, *Reverentially assisting with basic students' cognitive and spiritual learning needs as sacred acts, touching mindbodyspirit of spirit of other; sustaining students' human dignity*, is also relevant to the nursing education realm. Watson's (1979) older version of her ninth Carative Factor was often compared with Maslow's needs classification. However, in 2008, Watson discusses her ninth Caritas Process "within a context of what can be thought of as *Caritas Nursing* art/acts, or, more deeply, sacred arts of nursing" (p. 146). She further explains as follows:

> A *Caritas Nurse [Educator]* is conscious and aware of this perspective in assisting [the student] with basic [learning] needs, at whatever level of need is presenting. The nurse responds to these needs as a privilege, an honor, and a sacred act in assisting this [student]. The *Caritas Nurse [Educator]* appreciates that in this one act, he or she is connecting with and contributing both to the spirit of that [student] and to oneself." p. 147

Using this Teaching Caritas Process, nurse educators will, in partnership with students, identify their needs with the intention of providing the necessary assistance to facilitate their gratification, notably in relation to learning their future profession. In fact, satisfying students' needs will be most likely to help them reach a greater harmony as well as an enhanced quality of life at school. Guided by this Teaching Caritas Process, nurse educators are invited to respond to students' cognitive and spiritual learning needs as a sacred caring act to help and assist them in their apprenticeship of the profession. According to Watson (2008), the person may experience different needs. Some may be appropriate for teaching students. Table 6.2 shows Watson's adapted needs for students.

An example of students' needs could be associated with *academic achievement*: *self-efficacy*, *self-esteem*, and *self-concept*. Hence, guided by this ninth Teaching Caritas Process, nurse educators would realize the uniqueness of this need for each student. Indeed, Watson (2008) recommends working within the frame of reference of each person in order to appraise her or his specific achievement, in this case, academic achievement. The outcomes linked with this need are, as explained by Watson (2008), "self-approval, self-acceptance, and a level of competence and achievement that satisfies" the student (p. 176). Also, if nurse educators and classmates acknowledge the student's success and accomplishment, for example, during a laboratory activity, the student might be more likely to feel competent in the procedural skills.

Table 6.2 **Watson's Human Needs Exemplars and Their Adaptation for Nurse Educators**

Human Needs Exemplars	Students' Needs Exemplars
The need for work-purpose, contributing to something beyond self, something larger than self	The need to become a professional caring novice nurse contributing to humanity
The need for achievement—self-efficacy, self-esteem, self-concept	The need for academic achievement—self-efficacy, self-esteem, self-concept
The need for affiliation—family, love, and belonging	The need for affiliation—colleagues, educators, and belonging to the nursing school
The need for knowledge—understanding, making meaning (of life situation)	The need to integrate knowledge of the discipline and profession—cocreating meaning of the person's lived experience
The need for beauty-aesthetics	The need to understand the art of nursing and aesthetic knowing
The need for self-expression, creativity	The need for reflective practice, self-expression, and creativity
The need for play and relaxation	The need for play and relaxation
The need for an evolving self-actualization that is spiritually meaningful	The need for an evolving self-actualization within the nursing discipline that is spiritually meaningful with one's moral ideal

Source: Watson, J. (2008). *Nursing: The philosophy and science of caring* (Rev. ed., pp. 146–147). Boulder: University Press of Colorado.

Tenth Teaching Caritas Process

The tenth Teaching Caritas Process, *Opening to spiritual, mystery, unknowns—allowing for miracles to enter teaching/learning practices*, suggests nurse educators be open to the unknown within their nursing education praxis.

Watson (2008) proposes an existential–spiritual–phenomenological lens to better understand this perspective. This phenomenological lens invites nurse educators to better grasp their students' authentic learning experiences and meaning. In fact, Watson (2012) explains that phenomenology

> shifts the focus from facts and numbers alone to meaning, story, connections, understanding, and authentic expressions through a variety of creative scholarship: metaphor, poetry, art, music, drama, performance

or other forms that continue to evolve. Thus, new knowledge/understanding and language are revealed about a deeply human expressive phenomenon. (p. 99)

According to Cara's (1997) phenomenological methodology, entitled Relational Caring Inquiry, research participants are not viewed as mere subjects or objects to be examined and surveyed, but as coparticipants where the researcher embraces their uniqueness, wholeness, and human dignity. The openness, consciousness, and humanness originate from the relational caring ontology (Cara, 1997; Cara et al., 2017; O'Reilly & Cara, 2014).

Translated in the nursing education realm, nurse educators, guided by this Teaching Caritas Process, are invited to recognize their students' oneness through their journaling, narratives, or artistic creation. In doing so, nurse educators accompany them in the search for meaning associated with their individual lived experiences and learning journey. Moreover, this Teaching Caritas Process will help students feel understood in their apprenticeship on how to become a caring nurse.

Additionally, nurse educators inspired by this last Teaching Caritas Process, ontologically speaking, avoid preconceptions and judgments regarding students in difficulties. They rather remain open to miracles to enter their teaching/learning practices. In other words, nurse educators are encouraged to assist students while believing in their potential to succeed, not abandoning them but rather guiding them in finding strategies to attain the intended evaluation criteria for the class.

TIME OUT FOR REFLECTION

We invite you to write your reflection in a journal in order to link the preceding theoretical segment on Teaching Caritas Processes with your personal teaching/learning experiences.

Think about a time when you were in a situation where you could not help a student in need, and then ask yourself the following questions:

- How did you feel as a nurse educator?
- Which Teaching Caritas Processes could have made a difference for the student? And why?
- What could have been the student's outcome?
- Which three or four Teaching Caritas Processes resonate the most for you? And why?

PRAGMATIC SEGMENT
BEING INSPIRED BY THE TEACHING CARITAS PROCESSES
TO HUMANELY ACCOMPANY GRADUATE STUDENTS

Louise O'Reilly, PhD, MSc, RN, and Amélie Ouellet, MSc, RN

This story is twofold: first, the nurse educator's story and then the student's story. Both stories are necessary to exemplify the ways in which the Teaching Caritas Processes were used by the nurse educator and contributed to the student's learning experience.

The Nurse Educator's Story

From a Human Caring perspective, I have been aware, in my professional career, that "being with a person," whether in a state of illness or in another life situation, remains a relevant strategy to know, understand, and better accompany a human being. In my teaching functions, I had the privilege to supervise several graduate students, notably Amélie, from 2013 to 2018. During her master's program, Amélie was interested in exploring the nurses' ethical responsibility of advocacy toward adult patients living with intellectual disabilities and their families. I supervised Amélie along with a colleague, Professor Chantal Doré, from the School of Nursing at the Université de Sherbrooke, in Quebec, Canada. Our humanistic, respectful, individualized, and rigorous supervision, offered to Amélie throughout her graduate studies, has undoubtedly contributed to her academic success.

In the next paragraphs, I will examine, more closely, a specific moment experienced by Amélie and me, my teaching interventions as her supervisor, as well as the links between what I have achieved during this professorial guidance and the *Teaching Caritas Processes* (TCP). Following is my story.

To Listen and Understand Amélie's Lived Experience With Consciousness and Authentic Presence

In the summer of 2017, for a few months already, Amélie was concentrating her work on analyzing the verbatim of qualitative interviews done with the cared-for persons, family members, nurses, and managers.

In the fall of 2017, by email, Amélie informed us (both supervisors) of being "stuck" and of not knowing what to do to pursue the task in regard to this first experience of qualitative data analysis. She also mentioned being worried about not progressing in her analysis as expected in order to meet the deadline of her master's thesis submission (end of January 2018). When I received Amélie's email, I took the time to read and really understand the written content (related to the Watson's [2012] concept of authentic presence as well as TCP-2, TCP-3). In this caring moment, being conscious and authentically present (TCP-2), I did perceive, in this email, my student's anxiety and her important worries (TCP-3, TCP-5).

To Perceive Amélie as a Unique and Whole Human Being
As both a nurse educator and a graduate student supervisor, I came to realize that I accompany my students from a Human Caring perspective, leading me to perceive them as unique and whole human beings (TCP-3). By working regularly and closely with Amélie over the years, through an authentic and trusting relationship (TCP-4), I got to know her as a brilliant young woman, studious, organized, concerned to follow her supervisors' advice, and being able to plan and achieve her daily academic objectives (TCP-3). My regard for Amélie, filled with humanism (TCP-1), brings me to consider her as much more than a master's student. My regard is way beyond what is visible, by being specifically interested in the unique (considering Amélie's distinctive strengths and resources) and whole human being (considering both her personal and professional dimensions; TCP-3) that I have the honor to accompany her in her learning experiences and journey (TCP-4, TCP-7).

To Really Understand Amélie's Learning Experience
While reading Amélie's email, I associated in my head all the contextual elements that she described (her qualitative analysis not progressing to the anticipated rhythm, her being novice in qualitative research, her close deadline, as well as her anxiety) with her strengths (being organized, rigorous, and concerned to meet established objectives; TCP-6). By juxtaposing the contextual elements with her strengths

(TCP-6), I quickly realized that Amélie was experiencing a difficult learning experience (TCP-7) and that I needed (as supervisor) to respond and follow up, without delay, in order to meet her needs (TCP-6, TCP-9) and support and maintain her hope (TCP-2) during this particular academic moment, through an authentic and trustworthy caring relationship (TCP-4).

To Create a Safety Environment in Amélie's Learning Experience
In hope of supporting Amélie's learning (TCP-7) and a profound desire to help and assist her (TCP-1), a meeting was proposed as soon as possible in order to examine and discuss her work of data abstraction (in a table format) and its coherence with the verbatim collected during the qualitative interviews (TCP-6).

Seven days later, the meeting took place. Amélie had in hand paper copies of the results' tables and her laptop. Then, slowly and at her rhythm (TCP-1, TCP-7), I asked Amélie to share and explain her results so far and the links she had made between them and the research participants' verbatim collected during the interviews (TCP-5, TCP-7). The quality of our dialogue developed over the years (TCP-4, TCP-6) was a fundamental element in creating a safe environment (TCP-8) that allowed Amélie to express her anxiety, her questionings, her preoccupations, and her misunderstandings (TCP-5). The expression of her feelings and lived experience (TCP-5) were considered essential to enable learning (TCP-7) and rebuild her confidence in her own analytical abilities (TCP-2, TCP-3, TCP-9). Also, this safe environment (TCP-8) allowed me, as her supervisor, to ask questions in order to better understand her lived experience of analyzing the qualitative interviews in order to guide her toward accomplishing the data analysis (TCP-5, TCP-6, TCP-7).

At the end of our meeting, Amélie thanked me many times and mentioned that she did not know what she would have done if I had not been there for her to guide her throughout the process, restore her confidence in herself, and increase her motivation and hope in order to pursue and complete her data analysis (TCP-5). In this caring moment, I knew that my guidance had been helpful and meaningful and that I had adequately responded to her needs and concerns (TCP-9), contributed to believe in her potential for success (TCP-3) in order to regain hope (TCP-2). Overall, our caring moment brought more harmony in transforming this difficult moment into a rewarding and meaningful experience for her (TCP-10).

To Transform the Nurse Educator's Praxis Through Teaching Caritas Processes

In summary, as a nurse educator, to accompany, within a Humanistic Caring perspective, our graduate students corresponds to a moral ideal that I pursue. The Teaching Caritas Processes and their theoretical and humanist foundations remain exceptional guidance strategies to support us in our journey toward one's moral ideal as well as to deeply transform our pedagogical interventions, focusing, for example, on the establishment of a reciprocal, authentic, and trusting relationship with our students. Our renewed pedagogical interventions, inspired by the Teaching Caritas Processes, prove to be promising for the future, in offering a caring ontology for our professional practice toward our students.

The Student's Story

Amélie's Reflection, as a Nursing Graduate Student, of Being Supervised From a Human Caring Perspective

When I go back to that caring moment, where Professor O'Reilly accompanied me in my qualitative data analysis, I recall having experienced several feelings at the same time. Faced with this first experience of learning to do qualitative analysis, I remembered feeling insecurity and anxiety as well as being preoccupied with the lack of time to complete my master's thesis within the prescribed target date. These feelings were obstructive and limited me to move forward toward completion. Understanding my distress, Professor O'Reilly immediately invited me to meet with her in order to work together on my analysis.

When I sat down with her, I knew that she was really there to help me. I quickly felt understood, supported, and reassured. Her support was extremely significant in my journey, because I was able to understand how to proceed and make the necessary adjustments in my qualitative analysis. My nurse educator knew exactly how to share her scientific knowledge within a trusting and authentic relationship with me.

From her supervision, I was able to acquire a Human Caring perspective that still guides me in my professional work as well as in my personal life. I am convinced that this humanistic perspective comes from Professor O'Reilly, an important role model with whom I was fortunate to work. Indeed, she transmitted to me a vast scientific knowledge as well as a way of being that I have embodied during my apprenticeship, which made me a better person and a better nurse! Finally, her supervision has transformed me and allowed me, in turn, to become a humanistic–caring role model to my own students, through my teaching as a lecturer, and with my nursing colleagues, whom I encounter in my daily clinical practice.

CONCLUSION

Several clinical settings across the world are teaching Watson's *Clinical Caritas Processes* to their nurses to transform healthcare (Watson, 2018b). Diverse nursing schools worldwide also teach Watson's *Clinical Caritas Processes* to their students so that they can learn to become caring professionals in their future practice. However, being also informed by them in one's own teaching/learning practice with students can only attest that caring is indeed the "essence of nursing," and that not only in clinical practice but throughout various domains, in our case, nursing education. In other words, when nurse educators ground their teaching/learning practice on Human Caring, it makes the stance that caring for their students corresponds to their moral imperative.

To ground one's practice on the *Caritas Processes* does not only mean to teach them to students, but it implies to be informed and guided by them as well. In doing so, not only can nurse educators act as role models for their students, but it exemplifies the *coherence* and *unity* between what we know in terms of content (knowing), how we teach (doing), and who we are as teachers (being).

> This mode of *Caritas* thinking invites a total transformation of self and systems. . . . the changes occur not from the outer focus on systems but from that deep inner place within the creativity of the human spirit. Here is where the deep humanity, the individual heart and consciousness of [nurse educators], evolves and connects . . . and enters a more profound level of insight, personal/professional growth, understanding, and wisdom. (Watson, 2008, pp. 36–37)

Hence, this chapter intended to inform nurse educators on how to translate Watson's *Clinical Caritas Processes* into living *Teaching Caritas Processes* and how to be guided by them in their daily teaching/learning practices with their students. O'Reilly and Ouellet's Pragmatic Segment is helpful to exemplify the content of this chapter as well as witness its contribution to facilitate a graduate student's learning and accomplishment. Thus, the *Teaching Caritas Processes* can enlighten nurse educators to accompany their students in their learning journey as well as to develop caring relationships with their students in their praxis, contributing to humanize nursing education.

REFERENCES

Beck, C. T. (2001). Caring within nursing education: A metasynthesis. *Journal of Nursing Education, 40*(3), 101–109. doi:10.3928/0148-4834-20010301-04

Benner, P., Sutphen, M., Leonard, V., & Day, L. (2010). *Educating nurses: A call for radical transformation. The Carnegie report for the advancement of teaching.* San Francisco, CA: Jossey-Bass.

Bevis, E. O. (2000a). Teaching and learning: The key to education and professionalism. In E. O. Bevis & J. Watson (Eds.), *Toward a caring curriculum: A new pedagogy for nursing* (2nd ed., pp. 153–188). London, UK: Jones & Bartlett.

Bevis, E. O. (2000b). Teaching and learning: A practical commentary. In E. O. Bevis & J. Watson (Eds.), *Toward a caring curriculum: A new pedagogy for nursing* (2nd ed., pp. 217–259). London, UK: Jones & Bartlett.

Bevis, E. O., & Watson, J. (1989). *Toward a caring curriculum: A new pedagogy for nursing.* New York, NY: National League for Nursing Press.

Bevis, E. O., & Watson, J. (2000). *Toward a caring curriculum: A new pedagogy for nursing* (2nd ed.). London, UK: Jones & Bartlett.

Boykin, A., Touhy, T. A., & Smith, M. C. (2011). Evolution of a caring-based college of nursing. In M. Hills & J. Watson (Eds.), *Creating a Caring Science curriculum: An emancipatory pedagogy for nursing* (pp. 157–184). New York, NY: Springer Publishing Company.

Brown, L. P. (2011). Revisiting our roots: Caring in nursing curriculum design. *Nursing Education in Practice, 11*, 360–364. doi:10.1016/j.nepr.2011.03.007

Cara, C. (1997). *Managers' subjugation and empowerment of caring practices: A relational caring inquiry with staff nurses* (Doctoral dissertation). Retrieved from ProQuest Dissertations & Theses. (UMI No. 9728055).

Cara, C. (2001). The apprenticeship of caring. *International Journal of Human Caring, 5*(2), 33–41. doi:10.20467/1091-5710.5.2.33

Cara, C. (2003). A pragmatic view of Jean Watson's Caring Theory. *International Journal of Human Caring, 7*(3), 51–61. doi:10.20467/1091-5710.7.3.51

Cara, C. (2014). *L'école de pensée du caring comme pilier à la conception d'un programme de formation initiale en soins infirmiers: exemple québécois* [The Caring School of Thought as a pillar in the design of an initial training program in nursing]. Colloque multidisciplinaire, Institut et Haute école de la Santé La Source, Lausanne, Switzerland.

Cara, C., Gauvin-Lepage, J., Lefebvre, H., Létourneau, D., Alderson, M., Larue, C., . . . Mathieu, C. (2016). Le Modèle humaniste des soins infirmiers—UdeM: erspective novatrice et pragmatique [The Humanist Model of Nursing: Innovative and pragmatic perspective]. *Recherche en soins infirmiers, 125*, 20–31. doi:10.3917/rsi.125.0020

Cara, C., & Hills, M. (2018, May). *The added value of Caring Science: Its contributions to humanize nursing education.* Oral presentation at the Canadian Association of Schools in Nursing Conference, Montreal, QC, Canada.

Cara, C., Hills, M., & Watson, J. (2019). *An ontology of caring within nursing education: Re-imagining teaching-learning relationships with students.* Oral presentation at the International Association for Human Caring 40th Conference, Greenville, SC.

Cara, C., & O'Reilly, L. (2008). S'approprier la théorie du Human Caring de Jean Watson par la pratique reflexive lors d'une situation clinique [To acquire Jean Watson's Human Caring theory through reflexive practice in a clinical situation]. *Recherche en Soins Infirmiers, 95*, 37–45. doi:10.3917/rsi.095.0037

Cara, C., O'Reilly, L., & Brousseau, S. (2017). Relational caring inquiry: The added value of caring ontology in nursing research. In S. Lee, P. Palmieri, & J. Watson (Eds.), *Global advances in Human Caring literacy* (pp. 101–114). New York, NY: Springer Publishing Company.

Carper, B. A. (1978). Fundamental patterns of knowing in nursing. *Advances in Nursing Science, 1*(1), 13–23. doi:10.1097/00012272-197810000-00004

Caruso, E. M., Cisar, N., & Pipe, T. (2008). Creating a healing environment: An innovative educational approach for adopting Jean Watson's theory of Human Caring. *Nursing Administration Quarterly, 32*(2), 126–132. doi:10.1097/01. NAQ.0000314541.29241.14

Chan, Z. C., Tong, C. W., & Henderson, S. (2017). Power dynamics in the student-teacher relationship in clinical settings. *Nurse Education Today, 49*, 174–179. doi:10.1016/j.nedt.2016.11.026

Chinn, P. L., & Kramer, M. K. (2018). *Knowledge development in nursing theory and process* (10th ed.). St-Louis, MO: Elsevier.

Cook, P. R., & Cullen, J. A. (2003). Caring as an imperative for nursing education. *Nursing Education Perspective, 24*(4), 192–197.

Delmas, P., O'Reilly, L., Iglesias, K., Cara, C., & Burnier, M. (2016). Feasibility, acceptability and preliminary effects of an educational intervention to strengthen humanistic practice among haemodialysis nurses in the Canton of Vaud, Switzerland: A pilot study. *International Journal for Human Caring, 20*(1), 31–43. doi:10.20467/1091-5710.20.1.31

Falk Rafael, A. (2000). Watson's Philosophy, Science, and Theory of Human Caring as a conceptual framework for guiding community health nursing practice. *Advances in Nursing Science, 23*(2), 34–49. doi:10.1097/00012272-200012000-00005

Froneman, K., Du Plessis, E., & Koen, M. P. (2016). Effective educator-student relationships in nursing education to strengthen nursing students' resilience. *Curationis, 39*(1), 1595. doi:10.4102/curationis.v39i1.1595

Gillespie, M. (2005). Student–teacher connection: A place of possibility. *Journal of Advanced Nursing, 52*(2), 211–219. doi:10.1111/j.1365-2648.2005.03581.x

Goudreau, J., Pepin, J., Dubois, S., Boyer, L., Larue, C., & Legault, A. (2009). A second generation of the competency-based approach to nursing education. *International Journal of Nursing Education Scholarship, 1*(15), 1–15. doi:10.2202/1548-923X.1685

Halldorsdottir, S. (1990). The essential structure of a caring and uncaring encounter with a teacher: The perspective of the nursing student. In M. Leininger & J. Watson (Eds.), *The caring imperative in nursing education* (pp. 95–108). New York, NY: National League for Nursing Press.

Hills, M., & Cara, C. (2019). Curriculum development processes and pedagogical practices for advancing Caring Science literacy. In W. Rosa, S. Horton-Deutsch, & J. Watson (Eds.), *A handbook for Caring Science: Expanding the paradigm* (pp. 197–210). New York, NY: Springer Publishing Company.

Hills, M., & Watson, J. (2011). *Creating a Caring Science curriculum: An emancipatory pedagogy for nursing.* New York, NY: Springer Publishing Company.

Hughes, L. (1993). Peer group interactions and the students-perceived climate for caring. *Journal of Nursing Education, 32,* 78–83. doi:10.3928/0148-4834-19930201-09

Labrague, L. J., McEnroe-Petitte, D. M., Papathanasiou, I. V., Edet, O. B., & Arulappan, J. (2015). Impact of instructors' caring on students' perceptions of their own caring behaviors. *Journal of Nursing Scholarship, 47*(3), 1–9. doi:10.1111/jnu.12139

Murray, J. P. (2000). Making the connection: Teacher-student interactions and learning experiences. In E. O. Bevis & J. Watson (Eds.), *Toward a caring curriculum: A new pedagogy for nursing* (2nd ed., pp. 189–259). London, UK: Jones & Bartlett.

National League for Nursing. (2003). *Position statement. Innovation in nursing education: A call to reform.* Retrieved from http://www.nln.org/docs/default-source/about/archived-position-statements/innovation-in-nursing-education-a-call-to-reform-pdf.pdf

Noddings, N. (2012). The caring relation in teaching. *Oxford Review of Education, 38*(6), 771–781. doi:10.1080/03054985.2012.745047

Noddings, N. (2013). *Caring: A feminine approach to ethics and moral education* (2nd ed. updated). Berkeley: University of California Press.

O'Reilly, L., & Cara, C. (2014). La phénoménologie de Husserl [Husserl's phenomenology]. In M. Corbière & N. Larivière (Eds.), *Méthodes qualitatives, quantitatives et mixtes: Dans la recherche en sciences sociales, humaines et de la santé* [Qualitative, quantitative and mixed methods: In social, human and health sciences research] (pp. 29–50). Québec, QC, Canada: Presses de l'Université du Québec.

O'Reilly, L., Cara, C., & Delmas, P. (2016). Developing an educational intervention to strengthen the humanistic practices of hemodialysis nurses in Switzerland. *International Journal for Human Caring, 20*(1), 24–30. doi:10.20467/1091-5710-20.1.24

Payette, A., & Champagne, C. (1997). *Le groupe de Codéveloppment professionnel.* Québec, QC, Canada: Les Presses de l'Université du Québec.

Perry, A. G., & Cara, C. (2017). Explorer les fondements théoriques du caring dans la pratique infirmière (translation and scientific adaptation). In P. A. Potter, A.

G. Perry, P. A. Stockert, & A. M. Hall (Eds.), Soins infirmiers - Fondements généraux (4th ed., pp. 72–87). Montréal, QC, Canada: Chenelière Éducation.

Rockwood Lane, M., & Samuels, M. (2011). Introduction to caring as a pedagogical approach to nursing education. In M. Hills & J. Watson (Eds.), *Creating a Caring Science curriculum: An emancipatory pedagogy for nursing* (pp. 217–244). New York, NY: Springer Publishing Company.

Sitzman, K. (2016). Mindful communication for caring online. *Advances in Nursing Science, 39*(1), 38–47. doi:10.1097/ANS.0000000000000102

Sitzman, K., & Watson, J. (2014). *Caring Science, mindful practice: Implementing Watson's Human Caring theory.* New York, NY: Springer Publishing Company.

Touhy, T., & Boykin, A. (2008). Caring as the central domain in nursing education. *International Journal for Human Caring, 12*(2), 8–15. doi:10.20467/1091-5710.12.2.8

Watson, J. (n.d.). 10 Caritas processes®. *Watson Caring Science Institute.* Retrieved from https://www.watsoncaringscience.org/jean-bio/caring-science-theory/10-caritas-processes

Watson, J. (1979). *Nursing: The philosophy and science of caring.* Boulder: University Press of Colorado.

Watson, J. (1999). *Postmodern nursing and beyond.* Edinburgh, UK: Churchill Livingstone.

Watson, J. (2008). *Nursing: The philosophy and science of caring* (revised ed.). Boulder: University Press of Colorado.

Watson, J. (2012). *Human Caring Science: A theory of nursing* (2nd ed.). Sudbury, MA: Jones & Bartlett Learning.

Watson, J. (2017). Global advances in Human Caring literacy. In S. Lee, P. Palmieri, & J. Watson (Eds.), *Global advances in Human Caring literacy* (pp. 3–11). New York, NY: Springer Publishing Company.

Watson, J. (2018a). Reflection on teaching and sustaining Human Caring. In D. D. Hunt (Ed.), *The new nurse educator: Mastering academe* (2nd ed., pp. 189–194). New York, NY: Springer Publishing Company.

Watson, J. (2018b). *Unitary Caring Science: The philosophy and praxis of nursing.* Louisville: University of Colorado Press.

Whelan, J. (2017). The Caring Science imperative: A hallmark in nursing education. In S. Lee, P. Palmieri, & J. Watson (Eds.), *Global advances in Human Caring literacy* (pp. 33–42). New York, NY: Springer Publishing Company.

Wiklund-Gustin, L., & Wagner, L. (2013). The butterfly effect of caring—Clinical nursing teachers' understanding of self-compassion as a source to compassionate care. *Scandinavian Journal of Caring Science, 27,* 175–183. doi:10.1111/j.1471-6712.2012.01033.x

Habitus: An Ontological Space Fostering Humanistic Nursing Education

Colleen Maykut, DNP, MN, BScN, RN, and M. Carol Wild, MScN, RN

[There is a] strong and consistent concern to develop an ontology of care, a way of understanding ourselves not simply as doers and thinkers but as persons of care.
—Mercier, 1997, p. 3

LEARNING INTENTIONS

- Recognize how your personal and professional experiences as a nurse educator influence habitus to develop healing moments with students.

- Explore how the virtues of caring (wisdom, justice, and courage) are foundational for nursing education to nurture students' learning about health and healing.

- Appreciate the importance of healing, in nursing education, as the ontological mystery and structure of caring to ground students' future practice.

- Articulate the significant role of critical reflection in nursing education to foster our way of being to become caring nurse educators.

- Imagine, after reading this chapter's exemplar, a new way of being in relationship with your nursing students to nurture the next generation of healers.

INTRODUCTION

This chapter exemplifies how a caring worldview may enhance nurse educators' moral imperative to develop and foster "habitus," an ontological space, to enable students to explore healing as their professional purpose within a humanistic nursing education context. This ontological space is the "teaching moment" where the expressions of caring can be actualized between nursing student and educator. Embodiment, the actualization and expression of Human Caring, provides a foundational perspective for nurse educators, guiding them in the acquisition of the necessary knowledge, skills, attitudes, and attributes to foster humanistic education. Embodiment refers to the capacity and capability of nurse educators to harmoniously express the essence of their humanity grounded in Human Caring. Therefore, if embodiment is to be developed and nurtured, then knowing, doing, and being must be in harmony. This harmony enables the nurse educator to authentically create space for students to explore their future professional purpose and to understand the world they will inhabit (habitus). This habitus encourages self-integration as they both journey to self-transcendence (Roach, 2002).

First, the importance of understanding habitus as an intentional ontological space in which to authentically situate ourselves and speak and act justly in the world (our professional responsibility and accountability to be caring nurse educators) is considered. Second, both background and rationale for developing embodiment to create habitus as an ontological space for healing, being and becoming persons of care, is explored. This being and becoming is a critical aspect enabling nurse educators to wholeheartedly care for themselves and their students to promote healing as a fundamental expression of nursing. An exemplar will be provided in the Pragmatic Segment to illuminate these concepts through a student's eyes. Finally, throughout our discussion, reflective questions will be offered to stimulate readers to begin their journey of becoming caring nurse educators grounded in Human Caring.

AN ONTOLOGICAL SPACE WILL HELP US FLOURISH AS NURSE EDUCATORS

The dominant biomedical model reflects an illness and wellness dichotomy fostering a *us (healthcare professionals)* versus *them (clients)* mentality, reducing the individual to a label and creating a dehumanizing relationship (Cara, Nyberg, & Brousseau, 2011; Cowling, 2000; Ray & Turkel, 2014; Roach, 2002;

Turkel & Ray, 2004; Wright & Brajtman, 2018). The biomedical model, as a reductionist approach or a deficit model in the healthcare system, creates a situation where nurses, who practice deficit thinking, relinquish their humanistic caring (Hills & Watson, 2011). Unfortunately, best practice often is about survival and navigating structural processes with an emphasis on control, safety, compliance, risk consciousness, and standards, to ensure nursing students fit in and survive in the healthcare system. As nurse educators, we cannot let the *disease* totalize us, which systematically excludes the learning experience as we journey with our students.

This dominant perspective is also reflected by the adoption of a behaviorist paradigm in nursing education, focusing on measurement and competencies (Hills & Cara, 2019; Hills & Watson, 2011). Our current approach in nursing education is often to focus our academic energies on keeping up with technological advances necessary to work in the dominant biomedical paradigm (Ray & Turkel, 2014; Roach, 2002). As nurse educators and students, we cannot, nor should we, be separated from the world we dwell in, which informs our professional habitus. We need to utilize this life experience to foster authentic engagement with each other and thus embody our shared humanity (Picard, 1997). We have the ability and capacity to move toward freedom to restore and strengthen our personhood, as nurse educators. What we notice, what we care about, our skills, our values, our beliefs, and habits give us situated possibilities. We require existential skills of dwelling—the ability to embody experiences of meanings through our corporeal habitus (Babbitt, 2013; Benner, 2000; Simonsen, 2012). As nurse educators, we are moral beings and our actions are influenced by the places we inhabit, both personally and professionally (Austin, 2007). Therefore, it is vital that nurse educators understand how corporate structures influence choices we make in nursing education, such as "regulations, defined authority, written orders, ranks, incentives, punishments, formal task and occupational definitions, archetypal stories" (Musto, Rodney, & Vanderheide, 2015, p. 96). It is vital that we do not let a behaviorist paradigm prevent us from engaging in relational inquiry and practice with our students to create habitus and promote their health and healing perspectives. According to Hills and Watson (2011), an emancipatory paradigm shift, which embraces use of self, presence, and creation of shared space, is necessary in nursing education to promote learning and justice—reflecting our habitus. This habitus, which fosters embodiment, provides the ontological space for learners, both teachers and students, to flourish as persons of care while exploring health and healing as nursing's professional mandate.

Embodiment: Becoming Caring Nurse Educators

Human Caring is about conscious intention and action, a compassionate concern for humanity and has primacy for nursing (Roach, 2002; Roach & Maykut, 2010). Our actions are powered by our intentions, those energetic blueprints of what we believe is important, and thus potentials, both possibilities and capacities, are created (Watson, 2002). Embodiment is the actualization and then expression of Human Caring made visible in our practice; harmony of knowing, doing, and being. For nurse educators to express embodiment, they must have the necessary knowledge, skills, attitudes, and attributes to engage in critical reflection and scholarly development.

Embodiment is necessary for exploration of one's own beliefs and assumptions in the social context of the world we live in (Bourdieu, 1989). Nurse educators must engage in critical reflection (see also Chapter 3, Emancipatory Contributions to Humanize Nursing Education) and then discourse with peers to determine ethical and moral congruence between personal and professional perspectives for a harmonious life (Benner, 2000). This discourse in nursing education helps to situate ourselves in the present and envision the future while remembering our past. This engagement encourages us to evolve as we speak our multiple truths and cocreate shared meaning with our students.

Embodiment is about losing one's self as primacy—recognizing the importance of the student and the learning environment. As nurse educators, we must understand how contextual influences shape our decisions, desires, and actions becoming the pivotal opportunities for connecting with our students. Our essence, embodiment, is who we are, which is fluid and constantly evolving but always grounded in our identity as nurse educators. We must understand our corporal experiences in the world from a nondualistic and nondivisive perspective to invite students' stories to weave with our own, enriching the journey of our shared humanity within nursing education.

There is a paradox of being human and nurse educator; a questioning of where is home. Nurse educators are moored in the life of students—journeying together to discover a sense of personal belonging and professional purpose. This journey illuminates our shared humanity as we both consciously uncover and reflect on our own experiences. Being in relationship with our students is about letting go of self as primacy to become vulnerable (see also Chapter 5, Seeking Teaching/Learning Caring Relationships With Students). This vulnerability opens us to invite students into a human experience. When we speak of vulnerability, there is always a degree of risk involved. To be vulnerable is to espouse the virtues of caring, for example, wisdom, justice, and courage. "Wisdom," as reflected by our ethics, knowledge, and experience, enables us to enter into a caring relationship. As nurse educators, we require "justice" to best support students while navigating the boundaries necessary in a professional relationship. Finally, the "courage" to be free of expectations from students even when there may be disappointments and frustrations must be embraced by nurse educators.

Embodiment is about espousing the virtues of caring. Without embodiment there is a falseness of character. Nurse educators may say they embrace Human Caring, but their actions may not be congruent. For example, if a nurse educator believed in humanistic nursing education and a student requested an extension because of the death of a sibling, exploring options with the student would be a perfect example of Human Caring. The nurse educator would be interested in knowing how the student is coping, encouraging counseling through the educational institution if appropriate, and together deciding what type of extension would be in the best interest of the student to ensure success in the course. If instead, this nurse educator's response was to refer the student back to the course outline, which clearly states that no extensions would be granted, this would be an example of disharmony between what is believed and what is demonstrated. If Human Caring is harmony between knowing, doing, and being, then embodiment by nurse educators must be developed to ensure humanistic nursing education. Therefore, nurse educators must intentionally nurture habitus through our embodiment—harmony between our thoughts and actions, which is best supported through humanistic education.

Habitus: An Intentional, Inclusive, and Loving Space

Habitus is the space to create conditions to humanize nursing education. As nurse educators, we have a responsibility to bring "things" into "beings"—the shift from objectifying our students to valuing them as contributors in the educational relationship, allowing them to learn to focus on healing rather than curing. We also have a moral imperative to develop habitus to enable students to explore health and healing as their future professional purpose. It is a space where "shared meaning" through engagement in our teaching and learning relationships occurs (see also Chapter 5, Seeking Teaching/Learning Caring Relationships With Students); the opportunity for actualization of caring actions to foster healing moments. This space is vital offering inclusivity, appreciating and honoring differences, and flourishing to enable us to reach our potential as nurse educators and caring human beings. A space of justice created by learners, both students and nurse educators, serves as the premise for embodying a relational approach with self and others, inspired by love for humanity (McEwan, 2010; Roach, 2002; Roach & Maykut, 2010).

Cowling (2000) and Quinn (1997) suggest that the healing process is part of the human experience and is fostered when in relationship. Healing is not a dichotomous state of being healed or not healed but is irreducible, reflecting being in the "right relationship," suggesting congruency between aspects of our internal and external life (Quinn, 2000). Therefore, the nurse who is in the right relationship (embodiment) has the capacity and capability to develop habitus to foster healing, moving beyond the fixed binary prevalent in the biomedical model of illness–health. Healers "bring an authentic, caring presence and an open heart, a willingness to meet this other being as a unique, whole person with strengths rather than a set of problems to solve or a disease to cure. They bring love" (Quinn, 2000, p. 23). Relational willingness, embracing love (see also Chapter 4, Humanizing Nursing Education by Teaching From the Heart), risk, and vulnerability, creates openness to work within the space of "knowing" and "not knowing" and develops this embodied habitus. As Doane and Varcoe (2015) state, "to consciously consider what you know and what you do not know, how you relate as a knower, and to experience how a habit of knowing/not knowing can support more responsive and safe nursing practice" (pp. 28–29) is a critical part in developing a habit of conscious inquiry in students and nurse educators. It is within a loving embodied habitus that caring relationships can flourish. Sharing of narratives, between nurse educators and students, provides an opportunity to listen to another's story and brings context/insight into our own stories—creating an intentional, inclusive, and loving space. Nurse educators must be cognizant that narratives influence the learning experience, creating strengths and challenges, yet are foundational for developing authentic relationships and critical thinking.

Narratives, as opportunities for shared discovery of meaning between students and nurse educators, become a critical ethical space, an indivisible essence between self and others (Cowling, 2000; hooks, 1994; Latta & Buck, 2008; Quinn, 2000, 2010; Whitfield & Klug, 2004; Wright & Brajtman, 2018). This juncture, sacred space for shared meaning and connection, fostering self-reflection and enlightenment, becomes the birthplace of caring as relational—recognizing that meaning is always unfolding and never complete. There is ambiguity about who is being cared for and healed in the teacher–student relationship when viewed only from the nurse educator's assumed place of power and authority. For healing thoughts and actions to begin within nursing education there needs to be a human experience between students and nurse educators. Bevis and Watson (1989, 2000), Roach (2002), Hills and Watson (2011), as well as Hills and Cara (2019) suggested that caring theory is necessary to ground nursing education curricula and thus to provide the basis for relationship.

Embodiment, as harmony between an individual's actions and beliefs, being an authentic self, attracts others to engage in relationship through shared vulnerability. Embodiment begets healing energy when as nurse educators we recognize ourselves in our students. Human Caring keeps us in relationship by providing purpose and a sense of belonging (Roach, 2002; Roach & Maykut, 2010). That moment of habitus, experienced in learning moments, creates context for healing. When I am comfortable with myself, I am able to invite others to journey together—to experience both love and healing. Mutual respect and trust are foundational, but harmony must exist for embodiment to develop and thus create habitus. Therefore, Caring Praxis must be developed reciprocally, a humanist relationship between the nurse educator and the student to promote harmony, meaning, and dignity (Cara et al., 2016).

However, nurse educators need to remember we always come into the students' lives halfway through their stories and must understand their context. Within this shared context, an exchange of narratives enables nurse educators and students to engage in authentic relationships. This intentional act of sharing, with vulnerability, provides the opportunity to be seen and honored for who we are—an educational healing moment. It is the nurse educator's beliefs that begin to set the context for the initiation of this healing moment. Nurse educators who embrace healing are witnesses to suffering and can be guardians of hope by opening the sacred space: vulnerability. There must be congruency between *what we believe and what we do* as nurse educators to enable us to embrace vulnerability, which then becomes a pivotal moment to begin the learning journey of what it means to be a healer in nursing education.

Healing in nursing education is about creating space for students' authentic expression of their humanity, which is seen and honored by nurse educators. This acceptance of who the student is will enable them to be supported to reach their full potential (as future healers). We believe that everyone is whole—healing is about actualizing our full potential; we don't believe that we are broken and require fixing (curing)—healing is an ongoing process. We believe that the best way to understand and foster healing for the students' future practice is for them to be engaged in the process with the nurse educator, who must create the space for this unfolding of potential and actualization. Engagement in this process becomes easier when we perceive the universal humanity of another individual's suffering, which enables compassion to be revealed (Roach, 2002; Roach & Maykut, 2010). When compassion for self and others is revealed, habitus is actualized and a healing moment may occur. Healing as emancipatory creates conditions for students and nurse educators to experience the fullest expression of their freedom. A central perspective to ensure healing, foundational in nursing education, is to remember that wholeness always exists—we are already whole (Cowling, 2000). As nurse educators, it is imperative that we clarify the critical importance for students that healing is an expression of our shared humanity and must be embodied in their future practice.

Critical Reflection: Essential to Reach Embodiment for Habitus

> *It is through critical self-reflection that we become aware of why we attach the meanings we do to reality. . . . Reflexivity is a means to transform our understanding of the world we occupy and our place in it.*
> —Mezirow as paraphrased by Nairn, Chambers, Thompson, McGarry, and Chambers, 2012, p. 197

Reflection and developing as a reflective practitioner have been integral requirements for all professional groups in the 21st century (Kinsella, 2012). Within the creation of habitus, where sociopolitical and cultural influences on knowledge, skills, attitudes, and attributes need to be consciously understood and made intentional, critical reflection must be embraced by both nurse educators and students. In our view, reflection occurs primarily as an individual experience where our beliefs and values do not necessarily continue to evolve as there is no other to challenge our disposition. We believe to reach critical reflection, humanistic relationships in nursing education (among nurse educators or/and with students) must be developed to actualize the goals of professional learning and the development of habitus. By critical reflection, we mean a level of reflection or reflexivity where discourse between theory and practice (praxis) and a challenging of individual and system values occur.

Kinsella (2012) proposes a continuum of reflection and practitioner judgment. Her continuum has four stages: (a) receptive pre-reflection (intuitive/contemplative/aesthetic), (b) intentional reflection (reflecting in and on action), (c) embodied reflection (knowing how), and (d) critical reflexivity (discernment and interrogation of social conditions). Furthermore, she suggests that the stages are really dimensions of reflection, which are interrelated and joined through dialogic praxis. Kinsella (2012) offers an important distinction for us in understanding and interpreting reflection and reflexivity. As authors, we believe the last two stages, "embodied reflection" and "critical reflexivity," are the means to obtain embodiment to develop our professional habitus. In other words, engaging in critical reflexivity is ensuring the embodiment and creation of habitus by incorporating social and cultural influences, values, and beliefs. A reflective pedagogy is more than a model to be introduced to students to understand their professional habitus. It is about a way of thinking and processing information as well as challenging norms and conventions for change and progress—*becoming* a caring nurse educator to assist students develop their future professional purpose as healers.

TIME OUT FOR REFLECTION

Think about a recent teaching experience where you felt that you had been your very best in your role. Use your narrative to guide your exploration of the preceding concepts (habitus, embodiment, and healing) and we encourage you to recognize their expressions in your teaching practice. The intent of our guided questions is to sample dimensions of reflection, as suggested by Kinsella (2012). It takes time to embody a reflexive pedagogy and develop habitus.

"Habitus" is about *creating an ontological space*, a humanistic connection between student and teacher.

- How did you develop a humanistic connection with your students in your narrative?
- How would you describe your habitus grounded in embodiment and healing?
- Describe how the virtues of caring were exemplified in your narrative. How did your values and beliefs influence this teaching moment?

"Embodiment" is a *way of being caring*, situated in your understanding of your own habitus contextualized through the learning needs of students.

- Describe the values, attitudes, and behaviors which you embodied from a Human Caring perspective.
- What motivated your actions in the teaching relationship with the student(s)?
- What are the social consequences of embodying Human Caring in nursing education—for the student, the nurse educator, the patient, and ultimately the healthcare system?

"Healing" is about *creating space for a journey* of becoming and experiencing the fullest expression of our humanity.

- Has healing, as a concept, been part of your practice prior to reading this chapter?
- Describe how healing was actualized in your narrative.

- What could be the advantages of healing in nursing education, both for yourself and your students?

Reaching Critical Reflection. Now that you have completed your reflection, reread your journal and risk sharing it with another nurse educator. Remember, critical reflection includes a discussion with peers. Discuss how individual and system values influence your actions, ideas, and behaviors with respect to habitus, embodiment, and healing. How did you come to know and understand these new concepts?

CREATING HABITUS TO HUMANIZE NURSING EDUCATION

As nurse educators, we must embrace academic humility, leaving no room for hubris and power over. If we do not create this space for exploration and trial/failure/success, we will not prepare students to engage in practice settings where they feel comfortable, ready, and supported to embody their humanity. When an ontological space is created by the nurse educator, then students are able to discover what it means to be human and ultimately caring and healing nurses. Nurse educators must create moral habitability for learners to acquire the knowledge, skills, attitudes, and attributes to understand the practical work in which we are called to engage from a moral imperative.

Nursing's Habitus Grounded in Human Caring

As nurse educators, we have a moral imperative to foster embodiment, creating habitus reflective of and grounded in Human Caring. Creating this onto-logical space for embodiment and healing is the nurse educator's challenge. When we are comfortable within our own habitus, as a nurse educator and an intentional caring nurse, creating this space becomes more intuitive. We have educated our students to practice primarily within simple and compli-cated environments within a biomedical worldview (Hills & Watson, 2011). Therefore, nurse educators and students must understand how individual and system values influence their practice, especially in their role as healers.

Nursing students develop as "healers" by experiencing being cared for and heard by nurse educators in a habitus informed by Human Caring, which enables them to express who they are as persons of care. Our bodies have experiences that inform our habitus and influence the development of ontological space for relationships. As educators, we must foster an "embodied ethic" (Smith, 2012) to extend this space beyond the initial corporeal connection. Smith (2012) writes of a *pedagogy of intimacy for children* where caress enables a connection between two individuals, a critical moment of vulnerability, creating space to experience being cared for and loved through our bodies. Caress conveyed as physical, emotional, or spiritual by the nurse educator must be intentional during the teaching moment to authentically connect with students. A hand placed on a shoulder, a space to debrief after the death of a client, and acknowledgment of the student's uniqueness provide tangible actions as our shared humanity in this teaching relationship. Such examples allow us to see ourselves in others reinforcing our existence and purpose in relationship to students. A caress symbolizes our own vulnerability to enter and create this ontological space for a healing moment in nursing education. Many nurses are involved in creating habitus for healing. However, according to Jackson (2004), they do not recognize themselves in this role and are ill prepared from an educational perspective. Learning is not a means to an end but a journey about becoming, an actualization of one's self, and a freeing process of developing space for inclusive and ethical relationships to be fostered (Hase & Kenyon, 2007; hooks, 1994).

As nurse educators, we need to be sensitive to the context where our students will practice; ensuring they have the necessary knowledge, skills, attitudes, and attributes to engage as competent, ethical, moral, and compassionate nurses in a complex bureaucratic system. We have an ethic of responsibility to higher education, practice, and ultimately society. Creating habitus to humanize nursing education does not mean lowering standards. Competence, ethics and morality, and compassion are reflective of knowledge, skills, attitudes, and attributes, which are fundamental principles for nursing education (Roach, 2002). Instead of caring competing with *best practice*, Human Caring enables us to navigate using a virtue/value-based perspective to do the just act (Kagan, Smith, Cowling, & Chinn, 2009; Létourneau, Cara, & Goudreau, 2017; Ray & Turkel, 2014).

Becoming Besouled

We must bring our embodied knowledge as nurse educators, or as Picard (1997) suggests, becoming "besouled" to foster creativity in learning experiences. A besouled approach provides a lens for the nursing students to view the context (patient's life) instead of relying only on empirics or the objectification (the disease as a defining label). Being "besouled" is not just the integration of the mind, the body, and the spirit, but the belief, as Watson

(1999) explains, that they are not distinct but a unique expression of oneness, therefore best exemplified as "mindbodyspirit."

As nurse educators, we often teach students how to think and perform from a behavioral framework. Seldom do we teach or embody how to "be." How to "be" in relationship with patients and families taking into account their life experiences. How to "be" in relationship with colleagues, promoting collegiality. Finally, how to "be" aware of one's own life experiences shaping who students will become as healers. Embodiment provides the habitus for nurse educators and students to begin their journey of becoming "besouled" or as Watson (1999) suggests "being-in relation." Nurse educators must lead by example, embracing vulnerability, which means letting go of power and control as a context to develop and view the learning experience, as Hills and Watson (2011) have suggested. Instead, they must tap into the essence of who they are, their embodied knowledge, in which to design a learning relationship to foster creativity and, ultimately, acceptance of each other on a journey of becoming. When nurse educators and students are in relationship, taking into account each other's life experiences, they intentionally create space to accept and nurture each other. This ontological space provides an opportunity for a teaching caring moment in which healing may be expressed.

Attitudes and values, believing in one's potential, human dignity, liberty of choice, and moral engagement should be anchored in Caring (Roach, 2002; Roach & Maykut, 2010; see also Chapter 2, Educators' Caring Values, Attitudes, and Behaviors That Contribute to the Humanization of Nursing Education). In clinical contexts, caring encompasses the capacity of healing and curing; recognizing there is always potential to heal even when curing is not possible (Quinn, 1997; Watson, 2018). Human Caring focuses on persons and their experiences within the context of health and healing, to envision their horizon; "one's intentionality becomes activated through one's conscious focus towards aspects of reality that incorporate but transcend the physical as the object of attention" (Watson, 2002, p. 13). Human Caring, as descriptive language, allows for embodied intentionality to facilitate relational practice, wisdom, and rituals to guide nurse educators in developing ontological spaces for cocreating meaningful learning experiences with students. This embodied intentionality creates a common language to better express our human experiences in nursing education.

Latta and Buck (2008) mention that education needs to ground itself in an active inquiry approach utilizing our bodies to make meaning of knowledge separate from and also entangled with our body–world connection. As nurse educators, we must challenge our minds to explore the world in order to include corporeal experiences to help us better understand what it means to be human and besouled. As a discipline, we embrace the value of intellectualism at the expense of worldly and human understandings from a bodily perspective—we fear our body's ability to be objective. van Manen (1991) suggests that our relationships, for instance with our students, are the birthplace of empathy, compassion, and virtues, which enable us to engage in moral acts, and which, according to the authors, lead to embodiment and healing. Our actions, informed by ethics of caring, enable us to create space for the unfurling of a teaching caring moment, "recognizing teaching as a fundamentally situated, relational, and gestured encounter" (Smith, 2012, p. 65).

Therefore, healing moments in this ontological space must be experienced in nursing education, especially in undergraduate programs, to successfully instill this expression of Human Caring for the next generation of healers. Nurse educators must transform themselves to ensure they are able to care for students while ensuring the development of a caring habitus. This mindset embraced by nurse educators is not for their own goals and purpose but necessary for students, patients, and society; caring is offered without any expectation in return, or as Watson (2018) suggests, it becomes an altruistic expression of loving-kindness.

TIME OUT FOR REFLECTION

Think about a recent teaching experience which you felt was particularly significant for your understanding of becoming "besouled." The authors invite you to write your reflections in your journal to further link and reflect on the above theoretical segments within your personal teaching/learning journey.

- How did you utilize your academic humility (vulnerability and letting go) to accompany your students to learn about their future caring practice?
- Describe how "altruistic loving-kindness" and "becoming besouled" have been part of your teaching practice prior to reading this chapter.
- How has Human Caring language enabled you to develop this ontological space for unfurling caring–healing moments with students?

Reaching Critical Reflection. Now that you have completed your reflection, reread your journal and share your thoughts with another nurse educator. Remember, critical reflection includes a discussion with peers. Discuss how the concepts of academic humility, becoming besouled, and the language of Human Caring have influenced your actions, ideas, and behaviors. How did you come to know and understand these new concepts?

Offering Reflexive Courage

Our intent in this chapter has been to incorporate our experience about embodiment of caring to develop habitus. Our learning tells us that to develop a habitus requires critical reflection, being vulnerable, addressing power, embracing life experiences, and being open to both the known and unknown as they present in each experience. Utilizing Kinsella's (2012) continuum of reflection enables us to become besouled and thus, prevents us from thinking linearly and/or binary. Critical reflection has intensity and should be revisited often. As nurse educators, we invite you to take time to work through all stages on the continuum: to be pre-reflective, engage intentionally, nurture embodiment, and discern how individual and systems influence our nursing practice.

We also invite you to share with your students and enable them to see your reflexivity. Share with them your own learning and vulnerability. Reflect on your reflections, extend your understanding and being in your own becoming as a caring nurse educator. The Pragmatic Segment highlights the importance of critical reflection by a recent graduate's experience of caring teaching moments.

PRAGMATIC SEGMENT
LEARNING FROM CARING NURSE EDUCATORS:
HOW TO BECOME A HEALER

Cole Miller, BScN, RN

This exemplar will help readers grasp how a nurse educator's embodiment has been significant in developing habitus for fostering healing moments from a student's perspective. The creation of habitus enables students to explore healing as their professional purpose within a humanistic nursing education program. Students become healers when caring nurse educators inform, guide, and nurture them through meaningful learning experiences.

Humanistic Nursing Education: Formal Education and Informal Experiences "In the Margins"

As discussed earlier in this chapter, the biomedical model of care is often the dominant standard for undergraduate studies. Therefore, a nursing student is often struggling to balance the demand for a behavioristic "task-oriented" approach while attempting to foster a healing relationship with patients. Jackson (2004) as well as Watson (1999) both suggest that in addition to this model of "curing," it is imperative that we accept the idea of "healing," whereby nurses care for an individual holistically—mindbodyspirit. In order to achieve such a relationship, I agree with Hills and Cara (2019) as well as Hills and Watson (2011) that we need to explore the intimate act of caregiving in which the nursing student understands the importance of developing relational skills as vital to caring education. From my experience, providing excellent nursing care requires accepting the importance of embodiment along with its development and expansion through nursing education. Without this, we are unable to be open to and react appropriately to those for whom we care (Benner, 2000).

During my undergraduate nursing studies, I found that nursing education places a significant emphasis on the biomedical and quantitative style of teaching, diminishing the more qualitative art of nursing. Although not held at the highest importance, concepts of Human Caring were integrated into the curriculum in an attempt to solidify the foundation set out by nursing architects, such as Florence Nightingale, who utilized healing as a basis for her practice. Often, it is the margins, outside the formal teaching moments within the classroom or clinical setting, where we might experience this connection of caregiving from nurse educators. This connection provides the opportunity for a healing moment. My exemplar will explore the importance of humanistic education situated in the margins of my formal and informal learning.

Caring for Each Other

In the third year of my BScN program, I was asked to join a research group to study the phenomenon of men in nursing. The group was composed of a faculty member, an alumnus, and three current nursing students. This opportunity was "in the margins" because it was an extracurricular project which truly reflected the intimate act of caregiving. The nurse educator, whose teaching and scholarship are grounded in Human Caring, intentionally created a space to nurture and challenge the group members to flourish—as coresearchers and, ultimately, as healers. The faculty member trusted and valued our wisdom as men in nursing, which enabled us, as a group, to engage in meaningful relationships in a relatively short period of time as we cared for each other. As Cowling, Smith, and Watson (2008) explained, the act of caring itself addresses a level of wholeness corresponding to the essence of nursing, which in turn promotes healing. It is concepts such as these that have helped me to actualize my true potential in reaching a level of embodiment, balancing the biomedical model with Human Caring to acquire knowledge about becoming a caring nurse and healer.

Gaining Confidence as a Caring Nurse and Healer

Watson (2008) posits that the knowledge, connections, and relationships that we develop in Human Caring are fundamental to being/becoming caring as well as the very survival of humankind. As I reflect on my time in undergraduate studies, three years postgraduation, I realize that my journey as a caring professional was nurtured by nurse educators who embraced humanism. What these nurse educators had in common was compassion for self and others, the belief that being in a relationship supports professional growth for both the students and nurse educators, and recognizing the importance of creating a space for students to feel comfortable with acquiring knowledge, skills, attitudes, and attributes for their future practice.

Although caring content can be presented to students, it is sometimes the unplanned learning moments—in the margins—which demonstrate the relevance to the students of having a humanistic education grounded in Human Caring. I was introduced to several caring theories in a theoretical course; however, this knowledge became more meaningful to me with my involvement in the research study as a coinvestigator. Along with two other coinvestigators, we presented our findings at the International Association for Human Caring (IAHC) conference. I had never thought of having the confidence to deliver our results to an audience of Caring Scholars, but the nurse educator believed in our ability, as she sat in the audience. This ongoing belief and support by this nurse educator enabled me to present my fourth-year leadership project, the following year, as an oral presentation at the conference. My involvement with this association and the nurse educator's ongoing mentorship have provided me insights into a foundational way of being—nurse as healer. Although I had wholeheartedly embraced Human Caring as foundational for my practice, it was my involvement with and learning from this nurse educator and the said association that clarified the possibility of extending my practice to embody healing. These insights were further developed through discussions with peers, scholars, and mentors who challenged me to explore the notion of congruence in my practice. What I have come to believe about congruence is that both my actions and words are influenced by who I am as a person in this world and as a professional nurse. This life experience, grounded in critical reflection, becomes foundational for embodiment as a healer.

Embodiment and Reflective Practice

I have come to realize that to embody healing as a professional nurse, there are many aspects that need to be addressed. First, I must acquire the necessary knowledge of Human Caring to see the individual as a human being and not just the disease. Secondly, I must create a space for sharing narratives, which fosters understanding of the self and the other person. Thirdly, I must allow myself to be vulnerable for the unfolding of possibilities, which may intentionally create a space in which a caring moment may unfold for healing. I also realize the significance of having a community of like-minded mentors to support this ongoing growth as a healer. I believe it is essential that nurse educators increase the focus on creating meaningful learning experiences grounded in Human Caring with the ultimate goal of an integrated culture of healing. The connection formed between the student and nurse educator illustrated as transpersonal (see also Chapter 5, Seeking Teaching/Learning Caring Relationships With Students) and as presented earlier allows for a mutually valuable and dynamic relationship to develop (Watson, 2002). Fostering a caring relationship, which transcends the norm, must be a priority for nurse educators in order to nurture the next generation of healers.

Nurses as healers provide sacred space for a human experience to unfold and thus enable people to express their humanity. Likewise, nurse educators, as caring–healing teachers, provide sacred space for students' learning experiences of healing to unfold and thus enable students to express their humanity and their caring practice. I strongly believe that with an increased emphasis on blending Human Caring with health in nursing education, as suggested by Hills and Watson (2011), graduates will be able to embrace and articulate the importance of caring and healing in their future nursing practice. Although my exposure to the concept of healing began in university, I am consciously aware of the importance of nurturing my habitus, through my involvement in IAHC and my caring community, to embody and nurture myself as a caring nurse and healer. Embodiment is about becoming a person of care, grounded in Human Caring, and I recognize that healing, as my professional purpose, will be an ongoing journey.

CONCLUSION

Our intentions were to challenge your values and beliefs around the phenomena of embodiment and habitus as foundational for ensuring the art of healing as a mandate for nurse educators to be role models in their practice. Embodiment was proposed to situate the importance of embracing Human Caring to create habitus and healing, thus humanizing nursing education. This embodiment, although inherent in human beings, must be nurtured and role-modeled in nursing education. As nurse educators, we must exemplify these ways of caring in action as narratives and encourage our students to explore their capacity and capability to care and thus embody a healing habitus.

We view healing as the ontological mystery and structure of caring to ground students' future nursing practice. Healing is about fellowship; nourishing our humanity—the work of the soul in healing is about reflection, insight, and love (Roach, 2002). There is a need for evolution and growth of shared commitment with others in nursing education to facilitate learning about caring and healing for the self and humanity. Transforming each other and transforming together, we recognize healing is not linear, nor discriminatory — a space free of judgment, fostering inclusivity, and embracing and honoring difference. As nurse educators, we acknowledge our responsibility to ask questions, challenge the *status quo*, and develop as "moral agents" (Austin, 2007) and thus create habitus for healing in nursing education. We need to move beyond "teacher knows best (hubris) attitude" to recognize our privilege in being in relationship with our students (McEwan, 2010; Roach, 2002). We must recognize that the acquisition of disciplinary and practical knowledge is not enough to promote students' learning of a caring–healing practice. Students are longing, in their learning journey, for an ontological space where meaningful teaching/learning moments are created to foster the unfurling of their future professional praxis as healers.

Nursing students and educators must understand each other's professional lives and how they situate their personal and professional selves with the world—this will not only help them find their voice but begin embodiment and thus healing. All possibilities lie within the present moment (Cowling, 2000; Cowling et al., 2008), and nurse educators must be diligent in creating healing environments for our students as well as ourselves. We need to look for commonalities in our shared humanity. We should not decontextualize, generalize, or detach; rather we must embody mindfulness and acceptance of each other. Nursing education should be a haven, a habitus to develop capacity to demonstrate healing for self (while being nurtured) and others (through role-modeling) to learn and embody the nurse as healer.

So, why is healing a fundamental expression of nursing? Mayeroff (1971) believes it is the process of healing grounded in relationship that will enable us to evolve: "*I do not try to help the other grow in order to actualize myself, but by helping the other grow I do actualize myself*" (p. 40). As nurse educators, we have a moral and ethical imperative to create habitus for our students to foster their embodiment of caring, and as such, the opportunity to experience healing and prepare them for their future practice (Kagan et al., 2009).

We started this chapter with a quote reflecting the importance of understanding ourselves as persons of care. We would like to end this chapter with another quote to inspire you on your journey.

We cannot know caring unless we have learned it from within, for our self, with our self, and with others—within a relational worldview. Human caring begins with a love of self and other, of humanity and all living things—opening and welcoming the immanent and transcendent, the subtle, radiant, shadow-and-light vicissitudes of experiences of embodied living, dying, growing, changing, evolving; honoring with reverence the mystery, miracles, paradoxes, unknowns, the impermanence of changes while still actively, joyfully participating in all of it: the pain, the joy, and everything, believing in and allowing for miracles. (Watson, 2018, p. xvii)

Therefore, we need to move beyond "knowing" to "being." We must modernize Aristotle's phronesis as a context for understanding the self as healer. Settling into our personal place, our embodied habitus, is always remembering to turn inward to inform ourselves and then turn outward to illuminate others. We must embrace habitus as our ontological space to foster embodiment, which honors our ultimate expression of our humanity as nurses—*our way of being and becoming persons of care*. Embracing Human

Caring in nursing education informs and actualizes our nursing habitus, our home, in which to become a person of care who has the potential to create caring teaching moments for healing. As nurse educators, we are called to honor our lives as sacred, reach for the stars striving for our full-potential, and live virtuously—a professional and personal life actualized, essential for students' learning the nursing profession as future healers.

REFERENCES

Austin, W. (2007). The ethics of everyday practice: Healthcare environments as moral communities. *Advances in Nursing Science, 30*(1), 81–88. Retrieved from https://pdfs.semanticscholar.org/603b/e248e4f6cbdecc735beac4242d3f3cc0bd86.pdf

Babbitt, S. (2013). Humanism and embodiment: Remarks on cause and effect. *Hypatia, 28*(4), 733–748. doi:10.1111/hypa.12027

Benner, P. (2000). The roles of embodiment, emotion and lifeworld for rationality and agency in nursing practice. *Philosophy, 1*(1), 15–19. doi:10.1046/j.1466-769x.2000.00014.x

Bevis, E. O., & Watson, J. (1989). *Toward a caring curriculum: A new pedagogy for nursing*. New York, NY: National League for Nursing Press.

Bevis, E. O., & Watson, J. (2000). *Toward a caring curriculum: A new pedagogy for nursing* (2nd ed.). London, UK: Jones & Bartlett.

Bourdieu, P. (1989). Social space and symbolic power. *Sociological Theory, 7*(1), 14–25. doi:10.2307/202060

Cara, C., Nyberg, J. J., & Brousseau, S. (2011). Fostering the coexistence of caring philosophy and economics in today's health care system. *Nursing Administration Quarterly, 35*(1), 6–14. doi:10.1097/NAQ.Ob013e3182048c10

Cowling III, W. R. (2000). Healing as appreciating wholeness. *Advances in Nursing Sciences, 22*(3), 16–32. Retrieved from https://journals.lww.com/advancesinnursingscience/Abstract/2000/03000/Healing_as_Appreciating_Wholeness.3.aspx

Cowling III, W. R., Smith, M. C., & Watson, J. (2008). The power of wholeness, consciousness, and caring: A dialogue on nursing science, art, and healing. *Advances in Nursing Science, 31*(1), E41–E51. doi:10.1097/01.ANS.0000311535.11683.d1

Doane, G. H., & Varcoe, C. (2015). *How to nurse: Relational inquiry with individuals and families in changing health and health care contexts*. Philadelphia, PA: Wolters Kluwer.

Hase, S., & Kenyon, C. (2007). Heutagogy: A child of complexity theory. *Complicity: An International Journal of Complexity and Education, 4*(1), 111–119. Retrieved from http://citeseerx.ist.psu.edu/viewdoc/download?doi=10.1.1.397.5180&rep=rep1&type=pdf

Hills, M., & Cara, C. (2019). Curriculum development processes and pedagogical practices for advancing Caring Science literacy. In W. Rosa, S. Horton-Deutsch, & J. Watson (Eds.), *A handbook for Caring Science: Expanding the paradigm* (pp. 197–210). New York, NY: Springer Publishing Company.

Hills, M., & Watson, J. (2011). *Creating a Caring Science curriculum: An emancipatory pedagogy for nursing.* New York, NY: Springer Publishing Company.

hooks, b. (1994). *Teaching to transgress: Education as the practice of freedom.* New York, NY: Routledge.

Jackson, C. (2004). Healing ourselves, healing others: First in a series. *Holistic Nursing Practice, 18*(2), 67–81. doi:10.1097/00004650-200403000-00004

Kagan, P. N., Smith, M. C., Cowling III, W. R., & Chinn, P. L. (2009). A nursing manifesto: An emancipatory call for knowledge development, conscience, and praxis. *Nursing Philosophy, 11*(1), 67–85. doi:10.1111/j.1466-769X.2009.00422.x/full

Kinsella, E. A. (2012). Practitioner reflection and judgement as phronesis: A continuum of reflection and considerations for phronetic judgement. In E. A. Kinsella & A. Pitman (Eds.), *Phronesis as professional knowledge: Practical wisdom in the professions* (pp. 35–53). Rotterdam, the Netherlands: Sense Publishers.

Latta, M., & Buck, G. (2008). Enfleshing embodiment: 'Falling into trust' with body's role in teaching and learning. *Educational Philosophy and Theory, 40*(2), 315–329. doi:10.1111/j.1469-5812.2007.00333.x

Létourneau, D., Cara, C., & Goudreau, J. (2017). Humanizing nursing care: An analysis of caring theories through the lens of humanism. *International Journal for Human Caring, 21*(1), 32–40. doi:10.20467/1091-5710.21.1.32

Mayeroff, M. (1971). *On caring.* New York, NY: Harper & Row.

McEwan, H. (2010). Narrative reflection in the philosophy of teaching: Genealogies and portraits. *Journal of Philosophy of Education, 45*(1), 125–140. doi:10.1111/j.1467-9752.2010.00783.x

Mercier, R. A. (1997). Foreword. In M. S. Roach (Ed.), *Caring from the heart: The convergence of caring and spirituality* (pp. 1–3). Mahwah, NJ: Paulist Press.

Musto, L. C., Rodney, P. A., & Vanderheide, R. (2015). Toward interventions to address moral distress: Navigating structure and agency. *Nursing Ethics, 22*(1), 91–102. doi:10.1177/0969733014534879

Nairn, S., Chambers, D., Thompson, S., McGarry, J., & Chambers, K. (2012). Reflexivity and habitus: Opportunities and constraints on transformative learning. *Nursing Philosophy, 13*, 189–201. doi:10.1111/j.1466-769X.2011.00530.x

Picard, C. (1997). Embodied soul: The focus for nursing praxis. *Journal of Holistic Nursing, 15*(1), 41–53. doi:10.1177/089801019701500105

Quinn, J. F. (1997). Healing: A model for an integrative health care system. *Advance Practice Nursing Quarterly, 3*(1), 1–7. Retrieved from https://www.researchgate.net/publication/13745441_Healing_a_model_for_an_integrative_health_care_system

Quinn, J. F. (2000). The self as healer: Reflections from a nurse's journey. *AACN Advanced Critical Care, 11*(1), 17–26. Retrieved from https://aacnjournals.org/aacnacconline/article-abstract/11/1/17/13907/The-Self-as-Healer-Reflections-From-a-Nurse-s

Quinn, J. F. (2010). Habitats for healing: Healthy environments for health care's endangered species. *Beginnings (American Holistic Nurses Association), 30*(2), 10–11.

Retrieved from https://www.researchgate.net/publication/44627704_Habitats
_for_healing_healthy_environments_for_health_care%27s_endangered_species

Ray, M. A., & Turkel, M. C. (2014). Caring as emancipatory nursing praxis: The
theory of relational caring complexity. *Advances in Nursing Science, 37*(2), 132–146.
doi:10.1097/ANS.0000000000000024

Roach, M. S. (2002). *Caring, the human mode of being: A blueprint for the health professions* (2nd revised ed.). Ottawa, ON, Canada: Cambridge Health Alliance Press.

Roach, M. S., & Maykut, C. A. (2010). Comportment: A caring attribute in the
formation of an intentional practice. *International Journal for Human Caring,
14*(4), 22–26. doi:10.20467/1091-5710.14.4.22

Simonsen, K. (2012). In quest of a new humanism: Embodiment, experience and
phenomenology as critical geography. *Progress in Human Geography, 37*(1), 10–26.
doi:10.1177/0309132512467573

Smith, S. J. (2012). Caring caresses and the embodiment of good teaching. *Phenomenology & Practice, 6*(2), 65–83. Retrieved from https://journals.library.ualberta
.ca/pandpr/index.php/pandpr/article/view/19862/15388

Turkel, M. C., & Ray, M. A. (2004). Creating a caring practice environment through
self-renewal. *Nursing Administration Quarterly, 28*(4), 249–254. doi:10.1097/
00006216-200410000-00004

van Manen, M. (1991). *The tact of teaching.* New York: State University of New York
Press.

Watson, J. (1999). *Postmodern nursing and beyond.* Edinburgh, UK: Churchill Livingstone.

Watson, J. (2002). Intentionality and caring-healing consciousness: A practice of
transpersonal nursing. *Holistic Nursing Practice, 16*(4), 12–19. doi:10.1097/
00004650-200207000-00005

Watson, J. (2008). *Nursing: The philosophy and science of caring* (revised ed.). Boulder: University Press of Colorado.

Watson, J. (2018). *Unitary Caring Science: The philosophy and praxis of nursing.* Boulder: University Press of Colorado.

Whitfield, P. T., & Klug, B. J. (2004). Teacher as "healers": 21st century possibility? Or necessity. *Multicultural Perspectives, 6*(1), 43–50. doi:10.1207/
S15327892mcp0601_8

Wright, D., & Brajtman, S. (2018). Relational and embodied knowing: Nursing
ethics within the interprofessional team. *Nursing Ethics, 18*(1), 20–30. doi:10.1177/
096733010386165

8

Nurse Educators' Political Caring Literacy and Power to Promote Caring Relationships in Nursing Education

Sylvain Brousseau, PhD, MSc, BSN, RN, and Chantal Cara, PhD, RN, FAAN

> *To be influential, nurses must see themselves as professionals with the capacity and responsibility to influence current and future healthcare delivery systems. The nursing profession is based on the science of human health and the science of caring. It operates from a framework that values all people in a holistic way and seeks to foster and advance people's health throughout their lifespans and across all levels of society.*
> —Burke, 2016, para. 1

LEARNING INTENTIONS

- Understand how nurse educators' and school of nursing workforce's political caring literacy can contribute to humanize nursing education.
- Develop the ability to effectively understand how to politically influence nurse educators and school of nursing workforce to implement caring relationships in nursing education.

- Recognize how to identify your allies and use wisely the power and influence to create an environment where caring relationships in nursing education can flourish.
- Learn how to take advantage of the "game of politics" in order to implement and foster caring relationships within nursing education.

INTRODUCTION

This chapter aims to elucidate how nurse educators can influence politically their nursing school colleagues and workforce to shape the relationships within the institution. In order to implement Human Caring as a framework throughout the institution, we must know how to use humanistically our power of influence, aligned with political competencies and skills, with the nursing education administrators, nurse educators, and staff members. In doing so, this chapter intends to offer some political competencies, skills, and knowledge to the nurse educator community and nursing school workforce who want to humanize nursing education throughout their institution. This can foster and politically influence the team to implement humanistic relationships with their students, nurse educators, and staff members throughout the nursing school. This chapter ends with a Pragmatic Segment, followed by a conclusion.

POLITICS, POLICIES, AND POWER OF INFLUENCE: A NEW ARENA FOR NURSE EDUCATORS TO FOSTER CARING RELATIONSHIPS WITHIN THE SCHOOL OF NURSING ENVIRONMENT

Nurse educators make a difference in the lives of nursing students at the baccalaureate, master, and doctoral levels in nursing education. Nurse educators are often creative and have ideas that will favorably influence their nurse educator–students relationships (see Chapter 5, Seeking Teaching/ Learning Caring Relationships With Students). However, some improvement could also be done to humanize the school of nursing environment. Indeed, Duffy (2018), in her book called *Quality Caring Model in Nursing and Health System*, states about caring pedagogy that *"Caring*, as one of the core values of professional nursing, is honored, given high regard, and lived out through the behaviors of faculty members and staff in a school or work environment" (p. 258).

Like nurses from different domains of practice, we invite nurse educators to picture themselves as advocates improving quality, access, and engaging humanistic relationships within nursing education. Academic nurse educators should consider if and how nursing students are taught to be influential or future agents of change. Furthermore, focused efforts are needed at all levels of nursing education to prepare nurse educators to strategically assess political situations across educational policy levels and to adjust messages based on Caring Science. However, for many reasons, some educators may not know where to begin to implement and influence changes within their nursing school. They may need to learn by searching for evidence or completing research in political caring literacy or new pedagogical ways of teaching nursing, based on Human Caring, as a prerequisite to carry out this paradigm shift into nursing education.

In agreement with Patton, Zalon, and Ludwick (2019), evidence has shown that a strong foundation in policy led by nurses who are well grounded in political games has the potential to increase the policy competencies, in this case of a nurse educator. In other words, the key to success in making nurse educators' vision about caring relationships become reality is to deeply understand the policy-making process, being fully embedded in political actions and being strategic for a successful transformation within the nursing school. Grasping these political skills could help nurse educators become policy advocates to instill preferred changes within their nursing school. When doing so, nurse educators' caring vision could assist them in creating a humanistic influence among the nursing school workforce in order to invite each person to act from a Human Caring perspective to humanize nursing education.

The term *Politics* is defined as the use of relationships and power to gain ascendancy among competing stakeholders to influence policy and allocation of scarce resources (O'Grady, Mason, Hopkins Outlaw, & Gardner, 2016). In the domain of nursing education, Politics can be viewed as a process that requires nurse educators to become astute with both big *P* and a smaller *p* that we call politics. For Disch (2019, p. 331), *Politics*, with a capital *P*, is derived from the Greek word *politikos*, meaning "of citizens," "for citizens," or "relating to citizens." According to this author, generally speaking, *politics*, with a small *p*, is the ability of stakeholders (in our case, nurse educators, school administrators, and workforce members) to understand power relationships and contextual factors to act strategically to influence health spheres and health policy (in our case, nursing education). More specifically, politics refers to the skills and techniques used to run a government (Sonenberg, Leavitt, & Montalvo, 2016). Both definitions of

Politics and *politics* are applicable to all nursing domains, including education. Before describing the concept of policy, as it pertains to nursing education specifically, it is imperative to understand its general meaning from a Human Caring perspective.

Politics and Policy in Nursing Education: Using a Human Caring Lens

According to Ray and Turkel (2018) as well as Sonenberg et al. (2016), "policy" is defined as the deliberate course of action chosen by an individual or group to solve a problem. Policies exist at a unit (microsystem), institutional (i.e., nursing school), and societal level. Policies are elaborated through processes that are individually driven or collectively based. They can also address social issues within the nursing school, such as organizational effectiveness or pedagogical strategies. Up to this point, no consensus has been reached about the role of nurse educators in policy development and implementation at the levels cited earlier.

Moreover, for Ray and Turkel (2018), policy refers to "[p]atterns of energy and communicative actions associated with authority, power, control usually of leaders, administrators, and clinical staff" (para. 7). They add that "[p]olitical relates to hierarchical systems, roles and their differentiation or stratification, unions, and governmental influences that facilitate or challenge competition and cooperation in complex organizations" (para. 7). In addition, Brousseau (2018) declares that political nursing actions are essential to the practice of our profession, for example, to update our political nursing knowledge and exercise our social action role.

In the domain of education, a paradigmatic shift (Hills & Cara, 2019; Hills & Watson, 2011) into the nursing school institutions can be achieved only if nurse educators are relentless in pursuing their rightful place in policy skills, in partnership with the school of nursing workforce, by being committed and open to transform the environment into a caring education milieu. Nurse educators must advocate for students to experience nursing education based on a Human Caring perspective in order to become "humanist activists" in their future clinical, administrative, or teaching praxis. In agreement with Duffy (2018), such a political caring approach must start with nurse educators creating an environment based on Human Caring philosophy, facilitating students' learning and pointing out the "caring moment" grounded in teaching/learning caring relationships (see also Chapter 5, Seeking Teaching/Learning Caring Relationships With

Students). To accomplish that, nurse educators must be able to use their power of influence and political caring literacy in order to embrace and foster a caring philosophy within nursing education.

Power of Influence Within Nursing Education

PEACE powers arise from the power of love and the capacity to seek harmony in relationships with others. These powers are familiar in close family and friend relationships where the group requires ongoing cooperation and mutual support to survive as a group.
—Chinn, 2018, para. 4

According to Manojvlich (2007, p. 2), "powerless nurses are ineffective nurses." Most studies revealed that powerlessness is often related to several poor nursing outcomes, no matter the domains of practice, even in nursing education. Power is essential for political influence and to be able to make changes in nursing education, such as implementing a nursing undergraduate program inspired by Human Caring. Consequently, the widest and most informal definition of "power" is the practice of influencing other people, at an individual level (a colleague nurse educator) or at a broader level (the school of nursing as a whole).

Boykin, Schoenhofer, and Valentine (2014) claim that the development of an educational nursing program based on Caring Science acts as a global catalyst, a power of influence in itself to promote the universal visibility and significance of caring in nursing. It provides a global humanistic leadership for nursing education, clinical practice, and research grounded in Caring Science. For example, the nursing education program based on a caring approach often depicts the importance for students to learn various theories or philosophies of Human Caring, the essence of nursing. Such practice promotes the value of caring within our discipline (Boykin et al., 2014) and also influences the nursing school's mission, vision, and philosophy.

In other words, language can act as a power within the process of influence. Indeed, Watson (2017) argues that nurses should and must use a language associated with Caring Science Literacy in order to become part of a global perspective of health, healing, and human transformation. For example, Human Caring language can positively influence the school's administration to recognize nursing education's priorities related to relationships across educational practice and policies. To have an impact in policy circles, nurses need to learn how to construct strong arguments that translate caring perspectives into the institution's realities (Antrobus, 2004). However, influencing policies need more than the ability to gain access to the right political networks (despite its importance); it especially requires great capabilities to use the right language (Ferris, Treadway, Brouer, & Munyon, 2012). Montalvo (2015) also adds that there is a whole range of knowledge about political processes, lobbying, as well as various skills required to influence, which are not usually part of any nursing education undergraduate programs.

The "power of influence" means that there are opportunities to shape outcomes of a process, such as making a shift within the school of nursing to adopt a Human Caring perspective throughout its different nursing programs. Such transformation will not only influence the different courses to be taught in various nursing programs, but it will also influence positively relationships among administrators, nurse educators, staff, and students by its humanistic standpoint. In their day-to-day work, nurse educators especially influence students and other nursing colleagues. An example is when nurse educators support students working together on a class project to find solutions in their struggling relationships. Another example could be with other nurse educators, where one encourages a colleague receiving negative feedback from administrators about teaching evaluations. These are just a couple of examples of the complex relationships where nurse educators can exert their power of influence. The work of "influence" must be learned as one of the political skills that needs to be cultivated and owned much like the abilities and competencies used in working with nurse educators and other school of nursing members.

From our perspective, it seems that the potential of political power in the nurse educators' working environment has not been strongly recognized, and even less acknowledged. About unofficial power of influence, Disch (2019) states that "informal politics are carried out when we encourage colleagues to support a policy change at work, give an elevator speech to the [dean or the director of nursing school] about an initiative we are undertaking, or sit with the school of nursing member assembly at luncheon" (p. 331). There are numerous opportunities and ways to carry out informal politics and influence changes in an institution, such as implementing a Human Caring perspective throughout a nursing school. Inspired by Disch (2019), we outline (in Exhibit 8.1) some prerequisites and strategies useful to nurse educators to cocreate and embrace humanistic relationships based on Human Caring, within the school of nursing.

EXHIBIT 8.1 Prerequisites and Strategies for Nurse Educators to Cocreate and Embrace Caring Relationships Within the School of Nursing

CREATE ONE-ON-ONE OPPORTUNITIES TO DISCUSS AND MEET NURSING COLLEAGUES; GET TO KNOW BETTER THE NURSING SCHOOL MEMBERS

1. Attend an assembly meeting or a forum at work and discuss with someone you do not know.
2. Familiarize yourself with the school of nursing's mission, values, and strategic plan.
3. Identify your allies and nonallies within the school of nursing regarding a Human Caring perspective.
4. Invite colleagues for a coffee to gain their point of view on Watson's (2008, 2012, 2018) or Boykin and Schoenhofer's (2001, 2013) Human Caring theories.
5. Invite to lunch a colleague in disagreement to learn the person's point of view about implementing Human Caring in a nursing program.
6. Invite, for lunch or coffee breaks, administrators (e.g., the dean and vice-deans) to discuss their openness to a Human Caring approach as well as the feasibility of implementing such a perspective throughout the nursing school and in various nursing programs.
7. Take a coffee break with novice nurse educators in the first month of their arrival in the nursing school to share your ideas about Human Caring in nursing.
8. Make an appointment with the dean to share your ideas on how to cocreate caring relationships in the environment among nurse educators and team members.
9. Sit down with your colleagues and invite them to reflect upon the added value of Human Caring in the workplace.
10. Act as a caring role model with colleagues, staff, and students.
11. Join a professional nursing organization outside your work setting (e.g., The International Association for Human Caring or the Global Alliance for Human Caring Education).
12. Invite nurse educators to consult the websites of caring organizations, such as Watson's Caring Science Institute or Anne Boykin's Institute for the Advancement of Caring in Nursing.

13. Write a humanistic note to nurse educator colleagues to acknowledge their caring relationships in difficult situations, such as struggling to fail a student for ethical reasons or being in a complicated situation with a staff member.
14. Offer caring support to a colleague who is experiencing a conflicting situation.
15. Write a note/email to congratulate a clinical nursing supervisor for using a caring lens to resolve a difficult professional issue with a nursing student in a clinical setting.

EXPAND, SHARE, AND COMBINE BOTH YOUR CARING LENS AND POLITICAL KNOWLEDGE

16. Attend nursing or organizational congress based on Human Caring (e.g., International Association for Human Caring).
17. Participate in a Human Caring social networking group.
18. Become proficient with the school of nursing's mission, values, and strategic plan.
19. Subscribe to two nursing journals related to Human Caring and political skills.
20. Empower a caring workforce within the nursing school.
21. Invite a nursing scholar who is an expert on Human Caring and political skills to work with your nursing school to share innovative ideas on "political caring literacy."

Source: Inspired from Disch, J. (2019). Applying a nursing lens to shape policy. In R. M. Patton, M. L. Zalon, & R. Ludwick (Eds.), *Nurses making policy: From bedside to boardroom* (2nd ed., pp. 329–356). New York, NY: Springer Publishing Company.

TIME OUT FOR REFLECTION

We invite you to write your reflection in a journal to link the preceding theoretical segment with your own experiences regarding using your power of influence to cocreate an environment where caring relationships can flourish and be nurtured within your school of nursing.

Think about a situation where you felt that you had influenced nurse educators to be in caring relationships with colleagues or staff members in the workplace, and then ask yourself the following questions:

- Who were involved in the caring relationships within your school environment?
- What power strategies and skills did you use, as a nurse educator, to influence the caring relationships among colleagues and staff members?
- How did Human Caring inspire you to implement a caring relationship environment in your school?
- What were the advantages for yourself, your colleagues, staff members, and students?

FROM POLITICAL SKILLS TO POLITICAL CARING LITERACY

Nursing organizations and researchers need to take responsibility in supporting political skill development of the next cadre of leaders to enhance the personal and professional growth of leadership competencies. High level political skills are essential to enhance one's networking ability and interpersonal influence and to develop social capital to achieve both organizational and personal career goals.
—Montalvo and Byrne, 2016, p. 6

The Political Skills: Their Importance in Nursing Education

As explained by O'Grady et al. (2016) as well as Ferris et al. (2007), to be "politically skilled," you must be adequately prepared and qualified to perform a specific role. Moreover, it encompasses a combination of knowledge, skills, and behaviors that improve political performance. Politics surround us and is part of every organization—and nursing schools are no different. Nurse educators need to make the right political decisions if they are to succeed. They need to be able to identify the finer details of relationships, communication, and informal power structures within their nursing school. By accurately interpreting these different social situations, they can take action appropriately when the time comes and act as political role models for other colleagues. In addition, authors (Byrd et al., 2012; Staebler et al., 2017) insist that the political skills required for the exercise of political leadership be integrated into nursing education programs.

According to Vandenhouten, Malakar, Kubsch, Block, and Gallagher-Lepak (2011), "political leadership" is the ability of stakeholders (e.g.,

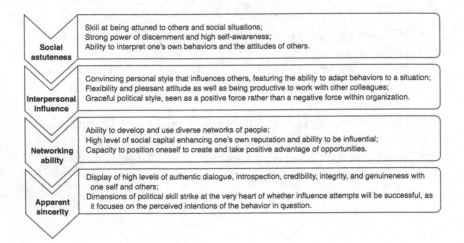

Figure 8.1 Essential elements to become a politically skilled nurse educator.
Source: Data from Ferris, G. R., Davidson, S. L., & Perrewé, P. L. (2005). *Political skill at work: Impact on work effectiveness* (pp. 9–12). Mountain View, CA: Davies-Black Publishing.

nurses) to understand power relations and contextual factors to act strategically in order to influence the professional, organizational, and public spheres along with health policies. A "political skill" refers to "the ability to effectively understand others at work, and to use such knowledge to influence others to act in ways that enhance one's personal and/or organizational objectives" (Ahearn, Ferris, Hochwarter, Douglas, & Ammeter, 2004, p. 311). These last-mentioned authors have also identified four elements characterizing political skills, which are important to keep in mind in order to gain political astuteness (see Figure 8.1). These elements (in Figure 8.1) are examples that could be used by nurse educators. However, readers have the opportunity to explore other elements that could inform their political skills.

Hence, we can ask the following question, How can nurse educators combine a Human Caring lens to their political skills? This question is discussed in the following section.

The Political Caring Literacy Model: Its Relevance for Nursing Education

The earlier mentioned political skills are aligned with Human Caring values (see Chapter 2, Educators' Caring Values, Attitudes, and Behaviors That

Contribute to the Humanization of Nursing Education) as nurse educators act from their humanistic ontological standpoint of being and becoming caring teachers (see Chapter 4, Humanizing Nursing Education by Teaching From the Heart), acknowledging their authentic presence in the moment, as well as the highest level of consciousness (see Chapter 3, Emancipatory Contributions to Humanize Nursing Education, and Chapter 7, Habitus: An Ontological Space Fostering Humanistic Nursing Education), both of which are essential to develop caring relationships (see Chapter 5, Seeking Teaching/Learning Caring Relationships With Students) within the school environment. In addition, in their political role, nurse educators must rely on an authentic dialogue and openness to be able to influence the school of nursing as a whole, its environment, including the relationships among administrators, colleagues, staff, and students. Consequently, a caring lens must underline the respect and uniqueness of all individuals, as well as the mutuality, trust, and equity throughout the relationships (among administrators, colleagues, staff, and students) taking place within the nursing education workplace.

According to Hills and Cara (2019), caring relationships in nursing education must be respectful, authentic, humanist, and based on credibility, integrity, sincerity, and genuineness. As also outlined in Chapter 2, Educators' Caring Values, Attitudes, and Behaviors That Contribute to the Humanization of Nursing Education, caring values and attitudes are relevant aspects of caring relationships in nursing education. Nurse educators must embrace their Human Caring literacy and their political skills along with their power of influence in order to move from a biomedical paradigm into a humanistic perspective, hence transforming the working environment to endorse Human Caring relationships across the nursing school.

Contrary to the common belief, nurse educators can have a profound influence with their colleagues to move toward adopting a Human Caring approach in their workplace, by using their political knowledge and skills to frame and define humanistic environment alternatives. In this context, we believe that influencing policy at different levels requires a strong set of caring values and attitudes combined with, what O'Grady and Johnson (2013) called, "sociopolitical knowledge," which corresponds to deep knowledge, political antennae, as well as power. Being inspired by O'Grady and Johnson's political knowledge model, we integrated a Human Caring Literacy perspective to cocreate a *Political Caring Literacy Model*, as an innovative reference to influence humanly and politically caring relationships across nursing education (see Figure 8.2).

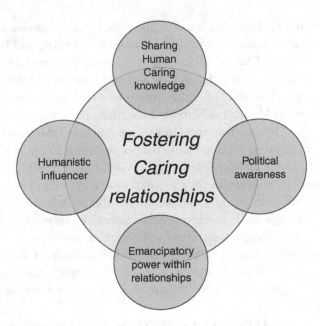

Figure 8.2 The Political Caring Literacy Model.

Before introducing the four components of our *Political Caring Literacy Model*, we want to remind nurse educators about the meaning of the word "literacy" (see also Chapter 6, Caritas Processes and Caritas Literacy as a Teaching Guide for Enlightened Nurse Educators). According to Hills and Cara (2019), the term "literacy" is "generally associated with the abilities to read and write but, in the Caring Science context, it has a more expansive meaning" (p. 197). Indeed, Watson (2017) clarifies the meaning of the term "literacy" as follows:

> [A] level of an expanded human consciousness: one who is able to access and process information, knowledge, images, and symbols, and to reflect, critique, interpret meaning—even construct and create meaning. Being literate extends to the ability to incorporate concrete experience, experiential learning, context, and situations into one's life field. Thus, the term *literacy* has evolved to reflect the fact that there are multiple literacies. . . . The vision of multiple literacies has opened the horizon to identify language literacy as an instrument of power and oppression—for example, considering dominant discourses and use of language—that endangers cultures and local knowledge. (p. 5)

Each of the four components of the *Political Caring Literacy Model* is discussed here. The first component of this new *Political Caring Literacy Model* relies on *sharing Human Caring knowledge*. It requires a mutual sharing of

Human Caring knowledge and expertise with colleagues. It involves know-ing our colleagues' perspective, including opposite views, in order to have a clear picture as well as sufficient information to support our standpoint and negotiate when needed. Being informed by the sociopolitical pattern of knowing, developed by White (1995), could be helpful to cocreate a Human Caring environment within the school of nursing, which appears, in itself, a major organizational challenge requiring a humanistic concerted action of all sociopolitical forces involved. Moreover, we suggest that nurse educators use a policy analysis framework, such as Hewison's work (2007), to help imple-ment policies, in our case, related to fostering caring relationships within the environment. For this to be achievable, nurse educators must acquire and link political and Human Caring knowledge. It will also help to grasp the strategic issues of negotiation and have a rigorous and structured agenda, giving a clear direction to humanize nursing education.

The second component is *political awareness*, which involves a global and continuous view of the working environment. It is critical that nurse educators consider not only their teaching colleagues but all personnel working within the nursing school. We invite nurse educators to remain flexible and consider other choices or scenarios to rally colleagues in work-ing together. Political awareness also requires active listening with policy-makers to understand their real motivations and develop strategies that fit the organization's political objectives (Kelly, 2014). If such reconciliation becomes inconceivable, it may very well entail the anticipation of possible ruptured relationships. This situation could seriously cause disharmony and harm, not only for the colleagues involved, such as nurse educators, but also to all the nursing school staff and perhaps even students. Hence, it might be advantageous for nurse educators to know the game of politics. In fact, Raso (2018) claims that the political game is "critical to success and key to navigating politics" (p. 1). She also adds that "[w]ithout diplomatic relation-ships and political capital, you won't achieve your agenda. You need allies, particularly those with influence" (p. 1). Nurse educators must be politically aware of their environment inside and outside their nursing school structure as government may impact the implementation and promotion of a caring relationship environment throughout the institution.

The third component refers to *emancipatory power within relationships.* This kind of power implies the ability to achieve a goal in the workplace, coherent with Human Caring, while pursuing emancipation of all colleagues involved within the relationships. In doing so, we believe that nurse educa-tors have a choice on how to use their power among team members within the school of nursing. Hills and Watson (2011) refer to the term *power with* rather than *power over.* They explain that there is reciprocity between power, knowledge, and control, and that, in order for there to be more equitable relationships, those with power need to give up and share control, so that others may benefit and share their knowledge, thus their power. Authentic power is shared power; it is power with, not power over. It does not negate faculty or nurses' responsibilities, skills or knowledge. It also means standing in one's own power, one's own truth and integrity, without succumbing to other's position of power, authoritarian control, and so on. (p. 17)

They go on to explain that "the power that leads us to our humanness is infinite. We have come to know that, the more of this type of power we share, the more we have returned to us" (Hills & Watson, 2011, p. 130). For Chinn (2018), using power is a choice that requires a noncondemnatory and a caring attitude at work. In the context of political arena, emancipatory power within a relationship is a power grounded on caring attitudes and values (see Chapter 2, Educators' Caring Values, Attitudes, and Behaviors That Contribute to the Humanization of Nursing Education). Concretely, it is being informed by caring values and attitudes, assisting nurse educators to influence positively each person within the relationships, and fostering, with dignity and respect, each other's professional emancipation. For example, a nurse educator could celebrate a colleague's success following a research project accepted for a national grant. We believe that this type of caring power of influence can only be supportive to achieve a humanistic transformation in nursing education.

The fourth component, *Humanistic influencer*, refers to nurse educators who are acting as caring role models, humanistic ambassadors to transform their workplace, freely sharing their expertise. Humanistic influencers can propose and support creative and innovative concrete solutions to solve relationship issues affecting negatively the work environment among administrators, staff members, and nurse educators in the school of nursing. To achieve a caring relationship environment, each person must apply his or her positive influence, and if possible, an emancipatory power within the organizational practices, grounded in a Human Caring lens. For example, nurse educators can approach their colleagues using a language coherent with Human Caring literacy (e.g., authenticity, altruism, dignity, integrity, and trust), which is more likely to promote caring relationships in the workplace. Another example could be a senior nurse educator who helps novice teachers find meaning related to their own future emancipation as assistant professors when being discouraged and ready to quit the nursing school.

TIME OUT FOR REFLECTION

We believe that these four components seek to *foster Caring relationships* in the nursing school. Such humanistic relationships should be embraced across the workplace in order to nurture a safe learning/teaching environment for all—administrators, nurse educators, staff members, and needless to say, students. Also, it can contribute to the development of a sense of belonging within the nursing education workforce. Finally, embracing the *Political Caring Literacy Model* could prove itself to be significant to implement caring relationships that will hopefully contribute to enhance nurse educators' personal well-being, professional satisfaction, and meaningfulness in one's daily learning/teaching praxis.

We invite you to write your reflection in a journal in order to link the preceding theoretical segment, pertaining to the *Political Caring Literacy Model*, with your own experiences, where you could have benefited from using an emancipatory power of influence to support caring relationships within your school of nursing.

Think about a situation where you felt that you could have better helped and supported one of your colleagues facing a challenge about relationships issues, then ask yourself the following questions:

- Can you share a significant experience regarding relationships issues among nurse educators in your nursing school?
- What happened? Who was involved?
- How did you feel about the situation?
- What are the facilitators and challenges that you met during this experience?
- Did you identify some advantages to be informed by the new *Political Caring Literacy Model* in this situation?
- Name two strategies based on the *Political Caring Literacy Model* that you could have used in this situation.
- What do you need to learn to be more effective in order to be inspired by the *Political Caring Literacy Model* to foster caring relationships and transform your nursing education workplace?

In the Pragmatic Segment, the experience of a director of undergraduate nursing programs exemplifies the importance of being informed by an emancipatory power of influence to work with nurse educator colleagues and staff to choose and implement a Human Caring philosophy that will foster caring relationships within the school of nursing.

PRAGMATIC SEGMENT
POLITICAL LIVED EXPERIENCES OF A DIRECTOR OF UNDERGRADUATE NURSING PROGRAMS FOSTERING CARING RELATIONSHIPS AMONG NURSE EDUCATOR COLLEAGUES

Sylvain Brousseau, PhD, MSc, BSN, RN

I illustrate how, as director of undergraduate nursing programs, I used my political influence and skills to implement a Caring philosophy (the *Nursing as Caring*, developed by Boykin and Schoenhofer, 2001, 2013), contributing to foster caring relationships within our work environment. In the period of 2017 to 2019, I implemented a new committee and invited administrators, nurse educators, and staff members in order to transform our nursing programs' philosophy. I therefore invited our school workforce to participate in a collective thinking, encouraging them to be creative and to share their innovative ideas to this paradigm shift in nursing education. The choice of *Nursing as Caring* originated from this committee.

Using Political Skills and Human Caring Literacy to Implement a Human Caring Philosophy Within the School of Nursing: The Director's Lived Experiences
As the director of two undergraduate nursing programs, I had responsibilities to accompany nurse educators in the implementation of the school's philosophy. Nurse educators also had a responsibility to participate in the process of this implementation.

My responsibilities were threefold:

1. To understand Boykin and Schoenhofer's caring philosophy in order to ground the structure of both undergraduate nursing programs in Human Caring Literacy

2. To develop and learn how to rely on Political skills, while combining Human Caring Literacy, to influence nurse educators to engage in this implementation process of transforming both undergraduate nursing programs' philosophy
3. To create opportunities (e.g., in formal and informal meetings and committees) in which each person (administrators, nurse educators, staff members) is involved in the process of being inspired by a humanistic caring philosophy in his or her day-to-day practice.

From my own experience, I strongly believed that translating Human Caring Literacy and Political skills implied sharing this knowledge with colleagues and staff members. Ultimately, using Human Caring Literacy combined with Political skills was one way to become a humanistic influencer toward nurse educators and staff members. Concretely, being informed by Boykin and Schoenhofer's work meant to manifest a caring leadership, rooted in connectedness, dialogue, authenticity, hopefulness, trust, humility, and courage. It also meant to bracket my own judgments and meet the person (administrators, nurse educators, staff members) as a unique human being with respect and dignity, acknowledging his or her full potential. These caring attitudes helped me to unify each colleague's perspective on how the school of nursing can be shaped in a way that our nursing education environment is grounded in the *Nursing as Caring* philosophy.

Moreover, this philosophy has been helpful, in my director's role, to promote caring relationships within the institution. In fact, Boykin and Schoenhofer (2001) recognize the importance of "personhood," to perceive each person as being unique and caring. According to them,

[p]ersonhood is the process of living grounded in caring. Personhood implies living out who we are, demonstrating congruence between beliefs and behaviors, and living the meaning of one's life. As a process, personhood acknowledges the person as having continuous potential for further tapping the current of caring. . . . This process is enhanced through participation in nurturing relationships with others. (Boykin & Schoenhofer, 2001, p. 4)

The Joint Venture of Caring and Politics to Be Successful in Implementing a Caring Philosophy Within the Nursing School

To succeed in this journey, as director, I needed to trust each person's goodwill to participate in the process. Additionally, nurse educators and staff members had to demonstrate openness and trust toward me. I also needed to make sure that the executive administrators of the university provided us with information regarding the university's mission, vision, and philosophy to implement a coherent transformation within our overall institution. During the transformation process, executive administrators had to show their commitment in our project by being our advocate, providing us with the necessary human and material resources, and demonstrating authenticity and honesty in their communication.

At the beginning, nurse educators were invited to engage in the process to transform the philosophy of their undergraduate nursing programs through a survey, individually having the opportunity to share their ideas and choices regarding an option that would be distinctive, representative, and inspiring for them. Nurse educators, who took part in the process of consultation, were able to identify some key themes (e.g., Human Caring, patterns of knowing, and social justice). The results of all of this work have led us to a consensus regarding the philosophical foundations to adopt in our nursing programs. For that to be successful, I tried to create a safe environment to share disagreements respectfully, openly, and in a constructive manner, without prejudice. At the end of this dialogical process, we decided together, to adopt, in a joint venture, the following underpinnings: *Nursing as caring* from the works of Boykin and Schoenhofer (2001, 2013), the *five patterns of knowing* developed by Chinn and Kramer (2018), as well as the *social justice* assumptions advanced by the Canadian Nurse Association (2010).

In a sense, both Human Caring Literacy and political knowing have not only provided me with knowledge but have also informed me as to *how* to accompany and influence humanistically the school's workforce throughout this transformative journey. In other words, this has fundamentally reshaped my way to humanely and politically influence changes in the school of nursing. Also, my learning endeavor was enriched by the partnership and the commitment of each person engaged in this philosophical transformation. I believe that everyone (i.e., administrators, nurse educators, staff members, along with students) can and will benefit from this new humanistic caring philosophy in our school. Indeed, such a change can only contribute to foster caring relationships within our environment, thus humanizing nursing education. Lastly, I invite nurse educators to use political skills in order to cocreate a collective consciousness group along with a stronger sense of belonging, hence promoting an authentic reflection and dialogue to renew their school of nursing's mission, values, and vision, rooted in Human Caring Literacy.

CONCLUSION

This chapter intended to inform nurse educators on how to influence politically and humanly in order to create a workplace (nursing school) where caring relationships are fostered among colleagues and staff members. While several authors have written about nursing and its involvement in policy, or lack thereof, this chapter is an innovative attempt to link Human Caring Literacy with the *politics and policy* knowledge within the domain of nursing education.

There seems to be an urgent need to provide nurse educators and nursing school staff members with Political literacy and skills, especially grounded in a Human Caring perspective. Being also inspired by O'Grady and Johnson's (2013) political knowledge model, a *Political Caring Literacy Model* was created to provide guidance to nurse educators to instill and enhance caring relationships in their workplace. We strongly believe that it is important to develop and preserve *caring relationships* among administrators, nurse educators, staff members, as well as students within the school of nursing to humanize nursing education. Lastly, we are convinced that political skills and an emancipatory power of influence rooted in humanism can only contribute to create a better environment for the future of nursing education as well as for the global nursing profession.

REFERENCES

Ahearn, K. K., Ferris, G. R., Hochwarter, W. A., Douglas, C., & Ammeter, A. P. (2004). Leader political skill and team performance. *Journal of Management, 30,* 309–327. doi:10.1016/j.jm.2003.01.004

Antrobus, S. (2004). Scaling the political ladder. *Nursing Management, 11*(7), 23–28. doi:10.7748/nm2004.11.11.7.23.c1999

Boykin, A., & Schoenhofer, S. (2001). *Nursing as caring: A model for transforming practice.* Sudbury, MA: Jones & Bartlett Publishers and National League for Nursing.

Boykin, A., & Schoenhofer, S. (2013). *Nursing as caring. A model for practice transforming.* Boston, MA: Jones & Bartlett.

Boykin, A., Schoenhofer, A., & Valentine, K. (2014). *Health care system transformation for nursing and health care leaders: Implementing a culture of caring.* New York, NY: Springer Publishing Company.

Brousseau, S. (2018). *Appel à la mobilisation: les infirmières en mode solutions. [Call to action: Nurses in solutions mode].* Retrieved from https://quebec.huffingtonpost.ca/sylvain-brousseau/appel-a-la-mobilisation-les-infirmieres-en-mode-solutions_a_23356706

Burke, S. (2016). *Influence through policy: Nurses have a unique role.* Retrieved from https://www.reflectionsonnursingleadership.org/commentary/more-commentary/Vol42_2_nurses-have-a-unique-role

Byrd, M. E., Costello, J., Gremel, K., Schwager, J., Blanchette, L., & Malloy, T. E. (2012). Political astuteness of baccalaureate nursing students following an active learning experience in health policy. *Public Health Nursing, 29,* 433–443. doi:10.1111/j.1525-1446.2012.01032.x

Canadian Nurse Association. (2010). *Social justice . . . a means to an end, an end in itself* (2nd ed). Ottawa, ON, Canada: Author. Retrieved from https://www.cna-aiic.ca/~/media/cna/page-content/pdf-en/social_justice_2010_e.pdf

Chinn, P. (2018). *Peace and power: A handbook of transformative group process* (online condensed edition). Retrieved from https://peaceandpowerblog.files.wordpress.com/2017/11/2018-handbook.pdf

Chinn, P. L., & Kramer, M. K. (2018). *Integrated theory and knowledge development in nursing* (10th ed.). St. Louis, MO: Mosby Elsevier.

Disch, J. (2019). Applying a nursing lens to shape policy. In R. M. Patton, M. L. Zalon, & R. Ludwick (Eds.), *Nurses making policy: From bedside to boardroom* (2nd ed., pp. 329–356). New York, NY: Springer Publishing Company.

Duffy, J. R. (2018). *Quality caring in nursing and health systems: Implications for clinicians, educators, and leaders* (3rd ed.). New York, NY: Springer Publishing Company.

Ferris, G. R., Davidson, S. L., & Perrewé, P. L. (2005). *Political skill at work: Impact on work effectiveness.* Mountain View, CA: Davies-Black Publishing.

Ferris, G. R., Treadway, D. C., Brouer, R. L., & Munyon, T. P. (2012). Political skill in the organizational sciences. In G. R. Ferris & D. C. Treadway (Eds.), *Politics in organizations: Theory and research considerations* (pp. 487–528). New York, NY: Routledge/Taylor & Francis.

Ferris, G. R., Treadway, D. C., Perrewé, P. L., Brouer, R. L., Douglas, C., & Lux, S. (2007). Political skill in organizations. *Journal of Management, 33,* 290–320. doi:10.1177/0149206307300813

Hewison, A. (2007). Policy analysis: A framework for nurse managers. *Journal of Nursing Management, 15*(7), 693–699. doi:10.1111/j.1365-2934.2006.00731.x

Hills, M., & Cara, C. (2019). Curriculum development processes and pedagogical practices for advancing Caring Science literacy. In W. Rosa, S. Horton-Deutsch, & J. Watson (Eds.), A *handbook for Caring Science: Expanding the paradigm* (pp. 197–210). New York, NY: Springer Publishing Company.

Hills, M., & Watson, J. (2011). *Creating a Caring Science curriculum: An emancipatory pedagogy for nursing.* New York, NY: Springer Publishing Company.

Kelly, K. (2014). Power, politics, and influence. In P. S. Yoder-Wise (Ed.), *Leading and managing in nursing* (5th revised ed., pp. 177–195). St. Louis, MO: Elsevier Mosby.

Manojvlich, M. (2007). Power and empowerment in nursing: Looking backward to inform the future. *The Online Journal of Issues in Nursing, 12*(1). Retrieved from http://ojin.nursingworld.org/MainMenuCategories/ANAMarketplace/ANAPeri odicals/OJIN/TableofContents/Volume122007/No1Jan07/LookingBackwardto InformtheFuture.html

Montalvo, W. (2015). Political skill and its relevance to nursing: An integrative review. *The Journal of Nursing Administration, 45*(7–8), 377–383. doi:10.1097/ NNA.0000000000000218

Montalvo, W., & Byrne, M. W. (2016). Mentoring nurses in political skill to navigate organizational politics. *Nursing Research and Practice, 2016*, 1–8. doi:10.1155/2016/3975634

O'Grady, E. T., & Johnson, J. (2013). Health policy issues in changing environments. In A. Hamric, C. Hanson, D. Way, & E. O'Grady (Eds.), *Advanced practice nursing: An integrative approach* (5th ed., pp. 579–606). St. Louis, MO: Elsevier Saunders.

O'Grady, E. T., Mason, D. J., Hopkins Outlaw, F., & Gardner, D. B. (2016). Frameworks for action in policy and politics. In D. J. Mason, D. B. Gardner, F. Hopkins Outlaw, & E. T. O'Grady (Eds.), *Policy and politics in nursing and health care* (7th ed., pp. 1–21). St. Louis, MO: Elsevier.

Patton, R. M., Zalon, M. L., & Ludwick, R. (2019). Leading the way in policy. In R. M. Patton, M. L. Zalon, & R. Ludwick (Eds.), *Nurses making policy: From bedside to boardroom* (2nd ed., pp. 3–35). New York, NY: Springer Publishing Company.

Raso, R. (2018). The game of politics. Editorial. *Nursing Management.* Retrieved from https://www.nursingcenter.com/wkhlrp/Handlers/articleContent.pdf?k ey=pdf_00006247-201803000-00001

Ray, M., & Turkel, M. (2018). Bureaucratic caring/transtheoretical evolution of Ray's Theory of Bureaucratic Caring [blog post]. *Nursology.* Retrieved from https:// nursology.net/nurse-theorists-and-their-work/rays-theory-of-bureaucratic -caring-transtheoretical-evolution-of-rays-theory-of-bureacratic-caring

Sonenberg, A., Leavitt, J. K., & Montalvo, W. (2016). Learning the ropes of policy, politics, and advocacy. In D. J. Mason, D. B. Gardner, F. Hopkins Outlaw, & E. T. O'Grady (Eds.), *Policy and politics in nursing and health care* (7th ed., pp. 38–48). St. Louis, MO: Elsevier.

Staebler, S., Campbell, J., Cornelius, P., Fallin-Bennett, A., Fry-Bowers, E., Kung, Y. M., . . . Miller, J. (2017). Policy and political advocacy: Comparison study of nursing faculty to determine current practices, perceptions, and barriers to teaching health policy. *Journal of Professional Nursing, 33*(5), 350–355. doi:10.1016/j.profnurs.2017.04.001

Vandenhouten, C. L., Malakar, C. L., Kubsch, S., Block, D. E., & Gallagher-Lepak, S. (2011). Political participation of registered nurses. *Policy, Politics & Nursing Practice, 12*(3), 159–167. doi:10.1177/1527154411425189

Watson, J. (2008). *Nursing: The philosophy and science of caring* (Rev. ed.). Boulder: University Press of Colorado.

Watson, J. (2012). *Human Caring Science: A theory of nursing* (2nd ed.). Sudbury, MA: Jones & Bartlett.

Watson, J. (2017). Global advances in Human Caring literacy. In S. Lee, P. Palmieri, & J. Watson (Eds.), *Global advances in Human Caring literacy* (pp. 3–11). New York, NY: Springer Publishing Company.

Watson, J. (2018). *Unitary Caring Science: The philosophy and science of praxis*. Boulder: University Press of Colorado.

White, J. (1995). Patterns of knowing: Review, critique, and update. *Advances in Nursing Science, 17*(4), 73–86. doi:10.1097/00012272-199506000-00007

9

Reflective Epilogue: *Being-Caring* Perspective of Teaching

This book offers a new lens and a new *Being-Caring perspective of teaching* as a new mandate for nursing education.

There is a hidden treasure in nursing education, which is often ignored: that is, the Being, the personhood, and vision of the nurse educator; that is, the consciousness, understanding, and wisdom, lived out in the classroom and outside the classroom. We must acknowledge and address the critical importance of the teacher and teaching itself. The philosophy and consciousness of the nurse educator, his or her beliefs, values, authentic presence, and responses/responsibility to those under the purview now requires attention. This transcends content expertise. This awakening is tied to humanistic ontological Ways-of-Being, as nurse educator and student, that intersect with learning, knowing, and doing. This shift addresses new global directions for society related to an emerging collective consciousness for humanity.

> [T]he 2017 Women's March for human rights that involved an estimated five-million people of all seven continents [is] a confirmation of the truth that we as humans have evolved to a greater awareness of the intrinsic worth and potential of each human life. [It is] evidence of a collective deep and conscious desire for a more just and [caring] peaceful society in which each of us can [fulfill] our purpose. (Milton & McCoy, 2017, p. 196)

This evidence of a more "collective deep and conscious desire for a more just and [caring] peaceful society in which each of us can [fulfill] our purpose" has profound implications for nursing, for teaching, and for us as nurse educators. We teach who we are. We practice who we are. We live out our lives' purposes by awakening to these global truths of valuing the intrinsic worth and potential of each human life.

There is a connection between a global collective emergence of "paying attention to intrinsic goodness of our shared humanity" and this emerging teaching perspective. In the world of education, we are called to shift our attention from the more corporate, industrial, authoritarian, didactic model of education to humanize teaching and learning—a call for honoring diversity, beauty, morality, and wholeness that appeals to higher instincts for an evolved, inspired civilization.

This global, collective emergence needed in teaching and learning has significant and enduring consequences for the discipline and profession of nursing and the next generations of practicing nurses, nursing scholarship, and nursing leadership for our world. One way forward is to focus our lens of "*Being-Caring*" as teacher and process of teaching.

BEING-CARING: A PERSPECTIVE OF TEACHING NURSING

What society needs at this point in history is "to break with the 'cotton wool' of habit, of mere routine, of automatism . . . to seek alternative ways of **Being** [emphasis added] . . . [t]o find such openings is to discover new possibilities—often new ways of achieving freedom" (Greene, 1988, p. 2).

The Spirit of Humanity is a global forum in which one of the authors (Dr. Jean Watson) was privileged to participate a few years ago. It "brings together leaders and practitioners who hold the view that the positive energy of love is the deepest, most enduring and most valuable characteristic of human nature" (Spirit of Humanity Forum, n.d., "What then is the true spirit of humanity?"). The aim of the forum was to identify and share ways of improving access to the inner strength of being. It emphasizes how love, compassion, and care for others can transform and truly rehumanize an institution (see Chapter 4, Humanizing Nursing Education by Teaching From the Heart). This aim is also related to caring as peace, as biogenic, as healthogenic, and as wholeness (Spirit of Humanity Forum, n.d.).

A professor once said, "You can get students to learn anything if it is done with love." This book reframes that as, "You can get students to learn anything if it is done with caring and love" (see Chapter 4, Humanizing

Nursing Education by Teaching From the Heart). This book addresses this void in the dominant discourse of nursing education, pedagogies, strategies, methodologies, technology, digital cyber-teaching, and so on. The Spirit of Humanity's more recent forum on *Peacefulness and Being Peace* noted: "As a new model for education emerges, *Being precedes Doing* [emphasis added]. Those who aspire to teach must constantly ask: 'Whom am I bringing to this encounter with the one I desire to teach?'" (Milton & McCoy, 2017, p. 199).

This *Being-Caring* perspective of teaching invites a self-awareness, a reflection, and a realization that "the teaching moment" can also be, and is, a "caring moment"; a "transpersonal caring moment" is an ontological turning point for teachers and students. It is honoring the mutuality of Being and Connecting while also creating a space-between, which can be expanded for a shared learning—a respectful giving and receiving that becomes part of complex patterns of our life, which informs our future and lasts a lifetime. Any nursing educational program and any educator of nursing are invited to address *Being-Caring* as teaching, addressing old and new evolving global teaching issues, for example, the teacher's values (see Chapter 2, Educators' Caring Values, Attitudes, and Behaviors That Contribute to the Humanization of Nursing Education); approach to student–educator relations (see Chapter 5, Seeking Teaching/Learning Caring Relationships With Students); and comfort with questioning, dialogue, vulnerability, encounter, challenge, and engagement.

Part of this teaching perspective of *Being-Caring* evokes and invites us to unlearn hierarchical teaching as well as learn to teach with critical consciousness and reflective praxis (see Chapter 3, Emancipatory Contributions to Humanize Nursing Education), with constructive ways of expressing feelings, humility, and being open to saying "I don't know. Let's learn this together." In *Being-Caring*, we apply Caritas (see Chapter 6, Caritas Processes and Caritas Literacy as a Teaching Guide for Enlightened Nurse Educators) in listening more closely to students, to hearing their feelings behind the words, to understand learning from the inside out; learning that teaching comes from inside the humanity of both nurse educator and student. This form of teaching/learning is an opportunity and privilege for unlimited creativity for shaping the future of nursing, of education, for an evolved human and a more civilized world and citizenry.

Being-Caring as teaching involves being grounded in a set of universal human values, of loving kindness, concern, social/moral justice, and Love of self and other, of humanity, and of Mother Earth (see Chapter 2, Educators' Caring Values, Attitudes, and Behaviors That Contribute to the Humanization of Nursing Education, and Chapter 4, Humanizing Nursing

Education by Teaching From the Heart). These are moral, humanistic values for human development, evolution of human consciousness for health, and well-being, evoking an ethic of belonging for a shared place for all in our world (Watson, 2018).

Being-Caring as Caritas Praxis

The focus on realizing one's full potential is a moral ethical concept, because honoring each person's opportunity for self-actualization enables universal values of Caritas, while making a connection between caring, love, peace, and nursing (see Chapter 2, Educators' Caring Values, Attitudes, and Behaviors That Contribute to the Humanization of Nursing Education; Chapter 4, Humanizing Nursing Education by Teaching From the Heart; and Chapter 6, Caritas Processes and Caritas Literacy as a Teaching Guide for Enlightened Nurse Educators). From a *Being-Caring* perspective of teaching, there is a oneness of Being/Doing/Knowing. This universal oneness, of teacher–student, of teaching/learning as one, is guided by ethical values, which serve as a guide for teaching nursing as Praxis—informed moral practice to live out caring, love, peace, and health through our *Being-Caring* as teachers in the world (see Chapter 2, Educators' Caring Values, Attitudes, and Behaviors That Contribute to the Humanization of Nursing Education; Chapter 4, Humanizing Nursing Education by Teaching From the Heart; and Chapter 5, Seeking Teaching/Learning Caring Relationships With Students). A *Being-Caring* teacher awakens to a collective and deep conscious desire for our profession and our society worldwide, to evolve to a moral community of caring—*Communitas* of Caring for our world (see Chapter 7, Habitus: An Ontological Space Fostering Humanistic Nursing Education, and Chapter 8, Nurse Educators' Political Caring Literacy and Power to Promote Caring Relationships in Nursing Education).

This *Being-Caring* perspective of teaching shifts from technical *knowing/doing* competency to *literacy*. This shift for *Being-Caring* translates to a Living *Eupraxis Teaching Nursing*—that is, practice of the good, the just, and the desire for more caring, compassion, love, and peace for our self, our profession, our humanity, and our universe.

Rhetorical Postscript

We are entering a new worldview, beyond the Western separatist ontology, to what Patti Lather (2017) claims is an "ontological turn" toward a cosmology that invites and welcomes the energy of these universal timeless values of caring, compassion, kindness, and Love back into our lives, our work, and our world. Lather asserts we need to be building a more socially just society. This requires critiquing the *status quo* and moves teaching as embodied *Being-Caring, as sacred activism* to fulfill nursing's covenant with humanity to sustain Human Caring (Watson, 2020).

To quote Greene (1978), the preeminent Teachers College educator of human freedom:

> The more fully engaged we are, the more we can look through other's eyes, the more richly individual we become. . . . [Teaching and] learning not only engage us in our own quests for answers and for meanings; they also serve to initiate us . . . into the human community . . . . Teachers who are alienated, passive, and unquestioning cannot make such initiations possible. (p. 3)

This *Being-Caring* requires Greene's (1978) "wide-awakeness" (p. 42), that is, a "wide-awakening"—a desire to ask moral-artistic, aesthetic questions of the world; a passion for teaching and radical learning, joys of living mindfully, of pursuing meanings as we live and learn. Greene's (1988) orientation of teaching/learning as tied to liberating human freedom is a form of "wide-awakened" sacred activism.

According to Harvey (2009), who coined the phrase "Sacred Activism,"

> Sacred Activism is a transforming force of compassion-in-action that is born of a fusion of deep spiritual knowledge, courage, love, and passion, with wise radical action in the world. The large-scale practice of Sacred Activism can become an essential force for preserving and healing the planet and its inhabitants.

Nursing and the public's need for sacred activism is awakened in the midst of proliferation of noncaring around the globe. This consciousness of sacred activism is evident with accelerating violence, dehumanization, bullying, hate crimes, and gun deaths, among other atrocities worldwide (Watson, 2020; see Chapter 1, Grounded in a Human Science Paradigm).

This ontological turn is entering into an ethical relational connection and covenant with students as coparticipants and equal partners (see Chapter 5, Seeking Teaching/Learning Caring Relationships With Students). The *Being-Caring* perspective honors the mutual commitment and inner life-world of each. There is an authentic attempt to capture the intersubjective relations and deep soul journey processes through shared coparticipation. Therefore, nurse educators and students are colearners and mutually engaged. *Being-Caring* teaching purposively *shifts from clinical teaching objectivity to authentic subjectivity/intersubjectivity*, mutual engagement, and human-to-human/spirit-to-spirit transpersonal connection. Space is created for a shared human connection. "Such thinking calls forth a sense of reverence and sacredness with regard to our [teaching], our lives, and all living things" (Watson, 2018, p. 46).

Thus, *teaching* and the *teacher* have an impact not only on learning but, perhaps more importantly, on the life-world and future of the students as well as the nurse educator (see also Chapter 7, Habitus: An Ontological Space Fostering Humanistic Nursing Education). Drawing upon the many years of experience, scholarship, and history of the authors and contributing scholars, this book opens a new window to Caring Science and its template as a guide for teaching, for the educators of nursing.

The *Being-Caring* perspective of teaching can determine whether the future professional nurse is awakened and equipped to enabling, preserving, and sustaining core humanistic values, a caring ethic, knowledge, human freedom, wisdom, and practices of human caring–healing and health for self and society. *Being-Caring* serves as the guide for *Caring Science* educators, for the next generation contributing to a moral caring community for inner and outer peace for our daily work and world.

REFERENCES

Greene, M. (1978). *Landscapes of learning*. New York, NY: Teachers College Press.

Greene, M. (1988). *The dialectic of freedom*. New York, NY: Teachers College Press.

Harvey, A. (2009). *What is sacred activism?* Retrieved from https://andrewharvey .net/sacred-activism/

Lather, P. (2017). *Post critical methodologies: The science possible after the critiques. The selected works of Patti Lather*. New York, NY: Routledge.

Milton, M. A., & McCoy, V. J. (2017). Being before doing: Transformation through an education for peace. In D. Cadman & S. Gill (Eds.), *Peacefulness: Being peace and making peace* (pp. 195–212). Reykjavik, Iceland: Spirit of Humanity Press.

Spirit of Humanity Forum. (n.d.). *Background*. Retrieved from https://www.sohforum .org/background/

Watson, J. (2018). *Unitary Caring Science: The philosophy and praxis of nursing*. Louisville: University Press of Colorado.

Watson, J. (2020). Nursing's global covenant with humanity—Unitary Caring Science as sacred activism. *Journal of Advanced Nursing, 76*(2), 699–704. doi:10.1111/ jan.13934

Index

standards of practice models, focus
on, 57
student–educator relationship, 2, 6,
9, 14, 23, 69, 75, 88, 118–119,
151. *See also* teaching/learning
caring relationships
added value for students and
nurse educators, 9–10, 96, 98
different constructs of, 88
humanist relationship, 145
knowing students as unique
individuals, 39–40, 75, 100,
131
positive/negative feelings,
expressions of, 119–120
promotion of mutual trust
within, 33–34, 41–42
shared context, 145
transpersonal caring relationship,
77, 90–93, 121–122, 155
students' learning, 23, 123
challenges, insufficient
acknowledgment of, 13–14
commitment to, 32–33, 41, 69,
122
critical dialogue, 124
experience
creation of safe environment for,
132–133
understanding, 131–132
influence of lack of humanistic
caring on, 12–16
lack of interest in, 14
process, presence in, 31–32
and reflective practice, 117
and respect, 25
rhythm/pace of, 77, 124–125
scholarly modalities pertaining
to, 123–124
and student–educator
relationship, 89

subjective inner life-world of self/
students, honoring, 115
success of students, lack of interest
in, 14

tacit knowledge, 55
teacher–student relationship. *See*
student–educator relationship
Teaching Caritas Process, 76–77,
109–111, 134–135
alternative pedagogical
strategies/ideas, 122–124
authentic presence, 114, 115,
130–131
being sensitive to self/students
by cultivating spiritual
practices, 116–117
caring–healing teaching/learning
process, use of, 120–121
compassion, 112
consciousness, 126, 130–131
enabling faith/hope/belief
system, 114–115
energetic authentic caring
educator–student presence,
environment for, 125–126
equanimity, 112
frame of reference of students,
staying within, 122
healing teaching/learning
environment, creation of,
125–126
honoring subjective inner, life-
world of self/students, 115
humanistic–altruistic values,
111–112
listening and understanding
students' lived experiences,
130–131
loving-kindness, 112, 113
miracles, 129

virtues of caring, espousing,
142–143
vulnerability, 70, 81, 120, 142, 145,
149, 150, 155

Watson, Jean, 78–79, 89–93,
108–109
wisdom, 142–143

Printed in the United States
by Baker & Taylor Publisher Services

Printed in the United States
by Baker & Taylor Publisher Services